UPSTREAM MEDICINE

DOCTORS FOR A HEALTHY SOCIETY

DOCTORS FOR A HEALTHY SOCIETY

UPSTREAM MEDICINE

FOREWORD BY DR VINCENT LAM

EDITED BY

ANDREW BRESNAHAN

MAHLI BRINDAMOUR

CHRISTOPHER CHARLES

RYAN MEILI

PURICH

Purich Publishing, an imprint of UBC Press
2029 West Mall
The University of British Columbia
Vancouver, BC, V6T 1Z2
www.ubcpress.ca

25 24 23 22 21 20 19 18 17 — 5 4 3 2 1

Printed in Canada from sustainable sources that are processed chlorine-and acid-free (interior pages 100% post-consumer recycled paper).

Library and Archives Canada Cataloguing in Publication
Upstream medicine : doctors for a healthy society / edited by Andrew Bresnahan, Mahli Brindamour, Christopher Vaughn Charles, and Ryan Meili.

Issued in print and electronic formats.

ISBN 978-1-895830-87-3 (softcover).--ISBN 978-1-895830-84-2 (PDF)

ISBN 978-1-895830-86-6 (Kindle).--ISBN 978-1-895830-88-0 (EPUB)

1. Social medicine--Canada. 2. Public health--Social aspects--Canada.

3. Health--Social aspects--Canada. 4. Physician and patient--Canada.

I. Bresnahan, Andrew, editor II. Brindamour, Mahli, editor III. Charles, Christopher Vaughn, editor IV. Meili, Ryan, 1975-, editor

RA418.3.C3U67 2017....362.10971....C2016-907523-0 ....C2016-907524-9

UBC Press gratefully acknowledges the financial support for our publishing program of the Government of Canada (through the Canada Book Fund), the Canada Council for the Arts, and the British Columbia Arts Council.

Printed and Bound in Canada by Houghton Boston Printers

Set in Minion Pro and ITC Kabel Std by Olson Information Design
Copy-editing by Karen Bolstad and Roberta Mitchell Coulter
Cover design by Olson Information Design

Funded by the Government of Canada
Financé par le gouvernement du Canada
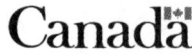

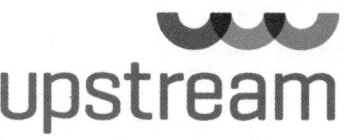

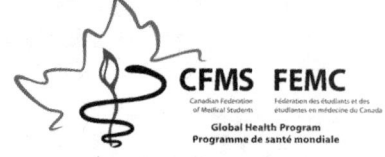

UPSTREAM MEDICINE - CONTENTS

▮▮ Foreword ▮▮

Dr Vincent Lam

As physicians caring for individual patients, we engage fundamentally in an act of imagination. We project our patients' symptoms, concerns, and predisposing risks into the possibilities that we call a differential diagnosis. Then, as clinicians, we recast the scenario before us, wondering how our treatments might divert an otherwise malignant progression of disease. Can we picture that a small antibiotic pill, which carries risks as well as benefits, might potentially alter the course of a potentially fatal pneumonia? Only our speculation of an alternate possible future for the patient in front of us makes any prescription humane and sensible. In treating patients, we must imagine helping them.

To think upstream about health is to broaden the scope of our imagination. It is to consider the roots of violence that led to a traumatic injury. It is to discern whether some gap in our society's emotional fabric has culminated in an addiction. It is to ask difficult questions: How have conflict and oppression, both within Canada and outside our borders, affected the patients for whom I care? Does an economic system that allows my patient to struggle for basic food and shelter impact their health in a drastic way? How do these forces affect my care of the individual patient? As a physician, what will be my response toward the injustice outside the walls of my clinic?

This is a collection of interviews by medical trainees, who seek to discern both their place in the medical profession and that of the profession within society. They probe the work of practising physicians who have decided not only to critically survey the world in which their patients live, but also to engage that world as part of their own deeply felt professional visions. Leaders in medicine from Canada's First Nations, physicians who practise amongst the traumatized and displaced both here and abroad, and physicians who have decided to enter government and politics; they are all upstream thinkers, who hope not only to swim in the river, but to change its flow for the better. Their levers for change come in a variety of shapes, sizes, and colours. The trainees wish to know: how can I help the patient in front of me within his or her reality? And then, can I imagine that this reality could be better?

This is a genuinely felt but complex aspiration. The science, the empirical evidence, and the details are important, as is the large vision for a healthier future upon this planet. By identifying biological mechanisms, and harnessing the focused applications of scientific process, stunning biomedical interventions have redefined our profession over the course of the last century. Meanwhile, we appreciate better than ever the crucial impact of factors as seemingly disparate as water security, political change, and childhood trauma upon community and individual health. Even as we are starting to employ gene therapy for cancers, we are beginning to understand that events external to an individual human being can influence the expression of his or her genome. The potential scope of an eyes-open, upstream perspective on health is therefore vast. It ranges from the macro to the molecular, from economics to the environment, encompassing politics and ethics. It is so large and interwoven that we are at risk of feeling that we cannot grapple with it effectively. More optimistically, we can hope to use the scope of current knowledge to reflect upon our collective wisdom, or sometimes lack thereof, and act with foresight and wisdom. These interviews concern the expression of this hope, where the personal meets the massive. They are portraits of individual physicians trying to simultaneously cherish the individual patient's dignity, while advocating for them on the large and sometimes harsh canvas of our unfolding world.

Always, it is about people – their dignity and humanity. The trainee asks: As physicians, what can we do for our patients? What is our most effective role in their broader life? Where can we push for good? We will always need the experienced, skilled clinician. Let us imagine an ankle expert. We would expect him to be very good at understanding and mending ankles. How useful if he observes how his patients' ankles are becoming broken and can find a way for this to occur less often. How profoundly useful if he knows where his patients need to walk.

To think upstream, we must fold into our own lives as doctors a radical type of imagination. This starts by understanding the patient in front of us, then the economic, political, and social forces that impact their health, and then daring to imagine and articulate future laws, systems, and ways of being that express our collective vision for health. As much as these questions provoke and inspire, they challenge us. So they must, as imagining health is nothing less than imagining a better world.

BRESNAHAN – BRINDAMOUR – CHARLES – MEILI

▬ Preface ▬

Andrew Bresnahan – Mahli Brindamour –
Christopher Charles – Ryan Meili

Staunching a bleeding wound or prescribing medications to alleviate a painful back may seem an adequate response in the isolated worlds of our doctors' offices and emergency rooms. But every clinical story is a social story, and each time patients present with acute medical problems or chronic diseases, they bring stories of the conditions in their everyday lives that made them sick in the first place. These stories about where they work, live, and play help us understand the "upstream" sources of what too often become complex, painful, and expensive health problems.

Thinking and acting upstream is a helpful metaphor: instead of standing downstream trying to save all those "drowning" people, why not also go upstream to find out why they fall in, and then work together to solve problems at their source?

A new generation of Canadian doctors is taking up this challenge. Armed with an understanding of what makes the biggest difference in the length and quality of our lives – the social determinants of health, including income, education, employment, housing, and food security – they are joining their patients and communities in a journey to improve the conditions of everyday life. They are digging for the roots of what makes people sick, and changing how we imagine the practice of medicine and politics in the process. They are building a healthier society.

Upstream Medicine features interviews with some of Canada's most celebrated health leaders by medical students and residents across the country, reflecting Canada's regional and linguistic diversity. Each interview explores a person and practice that brings evidence-based, upstream ideas to life. We learn the physicians' motivations for acting upstream, and of what is inspiring the next generation of upstream thinkers. Using personal stories and patient encounters to illuminate the social determinants of health and highlighting innovative solutions from across Canada, *Upstream Medicine* celebrates outstanding role models working to solve health problems at their source.

This project is the result of collaboration between Upstream, a non-partisan, non-profit organization based in Saskatchewan, and the Canadian Federation of Medical Students (CFMS), the representative voice of Canada's more than 9,000 medical students. Upstream is a movement that aims to build a healthy society through evidence-based, people-centered ideas. Combining the best available evidence on the social determinants of health with engaging storytelling, Upstream seeks to change the way we think about politics and health and to create space for decisions that will improve health outcomes for all Canadians. The CFMS is the voice of Canada's future doctors. It aims to bring global health and social medicine to the forefront of our medical community's preoccupations and contributes to the formation of future global health leaders.

This collection of interviews is more than the story of a few remarkable physicians. In these interviews, we wanted to shine a light on learners. There is a special relationship in medicine between people who are further in practice and those who are just starting on this path. That these busy leaders made time to speak to their junior colleagues about their efforts to achieve more justice and equity in health speaks of the power of the relationship between new learners and practising physicians. These discussions reminded our mentors of their initial dreams of making the world a better place, while showing future doctors that their idealism could indeed lead to making our world a healthier one.

As the editors of this collection, we were thrilled by the response from some of Canada's most celebrated physicians. When Joanne Liu humbly speaks to Claudel Pétrin-Desrosiers of the importance of keeping patients at the centre of our actions and fighting for them, as opposed to seeking personal advancement, they both remind us that today's medicine, in Dr Liu's words, is a social responsibility. When Ben Langer asks Meb Rashid about the patients who inspire him, we witness the way that the real struggles of real people drive physicians to push for policy change. When Jane Philpott, Canada's newest minister of health, tells her daughter Bethany, now a medical student at McMaster University, about how understanding inequities shaped her career, she reminds us how we can advocate upstream for people to live long and well.

The idea that social determinants and the wider environment have a huge role to play in health outcomes is not a new one, but it can be difficult to see how that understanding translates into a healthcare system so focused on clinical care and the response to illness. The upstream actions of the physicians profiled in this collection, whose work is made more pertinent through the eyes of those who will follow in their footsteps, gives us a glimpse of the types of leaders that can help us to build a better, healthier world.

▪▪ Chapter 1 ▪▪

Healthy Peoples and Healthy Discourse: Talking Indigenous Health

Evan Adams (First Nations Health Authority) – Ryan Giroux

I have had the good fortune to meet with Dr Evan Adams on a number of occasions, including at the inaugural Indigenous Health Conference in Toronto in 2014 as well as at annual gatherings of the Indigenous Physicians Association of Canada. Whether he is telling stories of growing up in the Sliammon First Nation of British Columbia or reminiscing on his time as an actor in an impressive number of feature films and television series, he is a captivating storyteller. On top of this, it is absolutely inspiring to hear him talking about Indigenous health, from individual patient interactions to tackling social determinants.

Not only does he have on-the-ground experience, but he has an impressive résumé, including completing a residency in Aboriginal Family Practice at the University of British Columbia, obtaining a Master of Public Health degree from Johns Hopkins University, and being the deputy provincial health officer for the BC government. Now Dr Adams has been named chief health officer of the First Nations Health Authority (FNHA), where he is responsible for leading a team that delivers health services to over 200,000 First Nations people throughout the province.

Dr Adams took the time to chat with me about his experiences in the many roles he has played over his career.

▥ **Ryan Giroux:** It's clear that the social determinants of health are an important part of your job as chief health officer for the FNHA in BC. What are some of the most prominent determinants that you have to consider in this role?

▥ **Evan Adams:** Well, there are the usual social determinants, and I think that you would probably get the standard answer that health outcomes are very directly related to one's educational outcomes, wealth, opportunity for employment, etc. However, for my clients (the First Nations people of BC), we look at other social determinants like culture and language, which are recognized by the United Nations as social determinants of Indigenous health. We also look at issues around social status. When we think of socio-economic status, we often think about it with a lot of emphasis on the economic part, like how poor or wealthy one is. I like to look at issues of social status as it pertains to race and racism as well as colonialism, given that Indigenous cultures are often non-dominant compared to settler cultures. The approximately eighty Indigenous cultures recognized by the UN are almost all within the territories of other nations, so those nations interfere with the ability of Indigenous people to self-determine, which itself is a factor in human health.

▥ **RG:** You used the phrase "social determinants of Indigenous health," which may be unfamiliar to some given that we are often taught about social determinants in general. Do you feel that physicians target these determinants across Canada and the healthcare system in general?

▥ **EA:** I think the healthcare system in general is overly focused on the individual's determinants of health because we are very focused on serving the individual client in the clinical fashion. We meet them, we talk about their medical histories, we examine them, we diagnose them, and we treat them. But if you ask a client, "What keeps you well?" they won't say, "Visiting with you as the doctor." They will say things like equity, equality, justice, fairness, and safety. They will even say things like beauty, love, and family – things that we have nothing to do with with us as doctors

It's quite hard for us to hold the fullness of the person's well-being in our minds and in our approaches. So things like having the basics, such as food, opportunity for education, housing, and basic safety – those are determinants of health for the vast majority of the population of the world. We take them for granted in Canada, and as clinicians, we are blind to the fullness of the person. It's hard for us to consider what role racism or oppression might play in in the well-being of my patient.

In medical school, you are learning to deal with a certain aspect of health and well-being: diagnosis and treatment. It's extremely important, but we also need to recognize that there are other aspects, and so I do worry when I speak to medical staff and they say, "Racism? That doesn't exist in Canada." It's a little bit short-sighted.

RG: I think we can agree that this is not the case, especially given some recent racism in healthcare reports. You were saying that culture and ethnicity are social determinants of Indigenous health, but there's a fair amount of confusion when it comes to thinking about these versus Indigeneity as a determinant. Do you perceive them to be different, and what are the differences if you do?

EA: Absolutely. Everyone has the potential to be an immigrant and to migrate. However, the concept of Indigenous peoples is that they are original peoples and, very often, the reality of an original people is that they are displaced; this is why an Indigenous person's situation is unique. An Indigenous person from Canada has a different reality of having their roots here for millennia and then being displaced by waves of migration that are fairly recent. On the other hand, an immigrant is someone who is here now and who uses resources to try and build a life. You'll hear that often from settlers; they'll say, "I came here with nothing – I have a special place in Canada." Our subversion of that as Indigenous peoples is that we've been here for hundreds of generations; we used to have everything and now we have next to nothing. It was the wealth of our territory that gave settlers their lives here. Our realities are different.

RG: Living on reserve and being First Nations yourself imposes this aspect of Indigeneity on your identity. I'm interested in hearing how you have seen the social determinants of health play out within your life and within your community.

EA: Well, I grew up with dozens of cousins who were exactly like me. I saw how they were sidelined by the educational system. I was a boy who could read a book, and I was overvalued for my ability to read and remember, whereas my cousins were undervalued for being strong athletic or strong traditional people. I had opportunity and I was given resources for an education, whereas they didn't finish grade twelve. They had limited opportunity for an education or work because of how they were sidelined so early. So many of my cousins are still there, whereas I had opportunity to move around, to be wealthy, to be well educated, to fulfill my potential, and to be happy. For them, maybe they didn't have as many options. First Nations people live on reserves not because they want to, but because they were put there.

Now one of the good things about our communities is that they are protective as well. My cousins, who were exactly like me, got to live in our culture, speak our language, and have a fulfilling life. But they also have to live with the other aspects that can shorten someone's life, like poverty and violence and disease. These things take a much larger toll on someone who hasn't been given the resources of someone who's educated, has money, is employed, and has knowledge. Having health knowledge and health literacy is protective.

RG: While it's evident that First Nations communities have health inequities, I really appreciate you acknowledging that these communities can also be positive and protective. It's very common to ignore the positives that can come from being Indigenous or being in a First Nations community. In terms of the healthcare system, policy-makers, governments, NGOs, and associated organizations, do you think they take too much of a negative approach when it comes to tackling Indigenous health issues?

EA: Yes, I think much of our business in health is a little bit reductionist and is focused on deficit. Much of our work as doctors is when someone is unwell as opposed to being well. We primarily give wellness back when it's been taken away, as opposed to contributing to the wellness of our communities.

As an Indigenous physician, I very much belong to a community and I provide health services to my own people. Because of this, I function in a different way – not in a transactional way, but in a community way. I'm supporting a community as opposed to being a clinician who interacts with a patient who is having a crisis. It's a different set-up and a different kind of interaction.

RG: Can you describe a time where the social determinants of health were illuminated in a patient interaction?

■■■ **EA:** I was always drawn to Indigenous populations, which is why I trained in medicine. Whenever I could see an Indigenous client, I would volunteer to go. I remember a few different patients.

One was an elderly gentleman who had been in residential school. I was proposing a very complicated course of medications that involved titrating a steroid daily that he had to adjust himself at home. In the middle of our meeting, he said, "Do you think I'm stupid? I know what you're saying." I could see that he was mistrustful of the medical establishment.

Another one was working in the Downtown Eastside of Vancouver with women in the sex trade. Very often people were scornful of them. There were many men – their customers – who were exploiting them. They would pay them, but hurt them. Other people around them said, "Ugh, those women. We don't bother with them – they're just whores and drug addicts." And we know that thousands of women are subjugated, oppressed, raped, even hunted and murdered, but we allow that in our society because we think, "Ugh, those are just bad women. They're so bad that we don't worry when they die." That's a horrendous collection of the social determinants of health where we essentially ditch very vulnerable women who are sick, poor, exploited, often uneducated, and often have mental health issues. We as privileged, wealthy, and educated people say, "We don't deal with this; we just deal with good people."

■■■ **RG:** How have these stories affected the way you practised medicine? Did it change the way that your career went, or the way that you saw patients or interacted with people?

■■■ **EA:** Well, actually, the experience of being with a poor patient was very normal to me because I'm from poor people. Those women in the Downtown Eastside – I could literally see them as my own sisters because they looked just like my sisters. They were women who were from places like I grew up in.

I actually learned a lot about inequity when I began working in government. When I was deputy provincial health officer for British Columbia, I could see how our 100,000 healthcare workers would pick and choose whom they helped. They would say, "We don't care about prisoners. We don't care about transgendered people and their health. We don't care about Aboriginal people – they're too complicated." We would constantly have to remind ourselves that we are the government: we have to look after everyone, not just the ones we like.

We can say, "I don't want to help girls, I don't want to help children, I don't want to help with abortions, I don't want to help with the poor or the coloured," and then we contribute to inequity. We must pledge to help everyone, even those who are hard to reach. That's a very difficult commitment to make, and most of us are not asked to make it. Most of us just say, "I'm only just going to help my section. I don't want those ones over there."

RG: Indigenous communities, whether they be First Nations, Métis, or Inuit, are traditionally focused on the community as opposed to the individual. It seems that you've taken these teachings and brought them into the way that you practise healthcare. Is that fair to say?

EA: Yes. One of our basic teachings is that the strongest hold up everyone, including the weakest, and no one gets left behind. If you and I are rich and we allow others to starve, then we are nothing. We are immoral people. We are disgusting people. We are not human

8

beings. A true Indigenous person will help all. It's a very painful and difficult topic – it's easy to say and hard to live.

Our goal is to be great human beings and not just to be great clinicians, and there's a difference. It's been well-proven that medical students lose their empathy over time. They lose their kindness and can become meaner. We must always fight that.

■■ **RG:** Thinking "upstream" is a helpful metaphor – instead of only standing downstream trying to help all those drowning in a river, why are we not heading upstream to find out why people fall in, and working together to solve problems at their source? How do you look upstream in your work?

■■ **EA:** One slightly different concern we have at FNHA is health literacy: the patients' knowledge of health and well-being. Do they know what good-quality foods are, not just do they have access to good-quality foods? Do they know why they need a mammogram after a particular age, or do they know how to get one? Do they know how easy birth control is to get? Do they know where to get a service, for example: "I have a growth or tumour or lump – where do I go to deal with that?" That's health knowledge. It is protective and saves lives, but we know that more highly educated people do better. For example, we know that if you took a group of young men and you watched which ones got HIV, you would see that young men who were less educated, had less money, had worse-paying jobs, and had less opportunity contracted HIV more frequently than the men who were wealthier, well educated, with good jobs, and lots of opportunity. It's been proven in hundreds of studies. At the FNHA, we are directly addressing issues of health knowledge to save people.

■■ **RG:** What steps do you think are important for someone to achieve adequate health literacy?

■■ **EA:** There are lots of ways to impart knowledge. One of them is to get knowledge to people when they're younger. Another is to do it in the language that they are speaking day-to-day. Another is to make it culturally relevant. So for instance, does Sesame Street speak to all cultures? Or does it speak to a particular culture? That's just an example of how you can make something meaningful or not meaningful to a learner.

Language within the healthcare system is quite important in the United States. The US has many people who don't speak English very well – they speak another mother tongue. The US system is much more responsive around translation and interpretation for patients. In Canada, we don't do it very well; we just expect people to speak English or French. When you're trying to explain the subtleties of resecting a tumour, you better have a darn good interpreter and not just be yelling at them in English.

I think that the Canadian healthcare system has a long way to go in serving its multicultural, pluralistic society. One of the ways we do it is by having a multicultural, pluralistic medical classroom. By just admitting the students with the highest marks without a thought to demographic representation, the system fails to serve the general population. Diversity within the classroom serves diversity within the country.

■■ **RG:** I'm the national officer of Indigenous health for the Canadian Federation of Medical Students, a new position developed in response to an increased need for mobilization on Indigenous health issues in Canadian medical schools. In that role, I've talked to a lot of medical students about Indigenous health, and there is a huge variation in knowledge of Indigenous people and health among medical students, who eventually go on to contribute to variation within the field of medicine. What variation have you seen in the field of medicine or in larger policy-making bodies that you're involved in?

EA: In the 1990s when I was training, some of my older colleagues were still marvelling at the feminization of the workforce. They remembered a time when all the doctors were men. To them, they couldn't believe it – with all these women now, everything was so different. Times do change, so I think now it is better for us as Indigenous physicians and as Indigenous medical students. I hope that our classmates and colleagues are more tolerant, that they understand diversity or the need for it, and that they have some cultural competence. My sense and my hope is that we're nurturing that cultural competence better than when I was in the medical classroom.

RG: A reflective practice is one of the hallmarks of cultural safety as opposed to cultural competence: not to just acknowledge your own privilege or differences in culture, but to reflect on it and see how you can make somebody's healthcare interaction best for them. We've consistently seen report after report of racism and cultural incompetency within the healthcare system in Canada. It's a very pervasive system we have here and it seems that often Indigenous people don't have culturally safe healthcare interactions. How do we start reversing this?

EA: First of all, we can acknowledge that sometimes when a patient of colour has a bad outcome, that sometimes it's because of institutional or practitioner factors. That's actually really hard, I think, for most of the people in our trade to acknowledge – that racism exists and that clinician bias exists. Clinician bias was really well described in "First Peoples, Second Class Treatment" [a report on racism toward Indigenous peoples in the Canadian healthcare system], and it exposes that clinician bias can play a role in a bad outcome. A clinician can make a decision not to treat a client to the standard because they think that the patient isn't quite deserving of that standard of treatment. You will see that many places will say, "No, racism doesn't exist on my ward; none of my doctors are careless," and that there is no room for improvement or that they're perfect the way they are. It's really an odd posture. There is a need for changing leadership that says that says, "look, we can make things better."

The second step is to lead change, and the third is to be the change. Let's make changes to make a safe environment for all our clients. Let's speak to clinicians so they understand that the goal is to have a respectful encounter 100 per cent of the time and make sure that our health outcomes are exactly the same. For example, researchers saw that transplant rates between African-Americans and Caucasian-Americans were different, even when they controlled for other factors. There's a bias toward giving white people kidneys and taking care of them very well, and a bias against African-Americans to not give them transplants and not follow up with the best care possible.

RG: You've said that we need to acknowledge and then move forward in being the change in this issue, but one of the issues is that there have been many funding constraints for non-governmental Indigenous health organizations. For example, the National Aboriginal Health Organization is now defunct because of a lack of federal funding. How do we adequately mobilize on these issues given the lack of funding to these larger organizations? What kind of political environment would be ideal to improve Indigenous health in Canada?

EA: I think it's safe to say that sometimes health policy decisions are driven by ideology rather than evidence. You can have situations like "We don't give opioids to drug users because we don't like the idea of government giving heroin for free to drug addicts," even when the evidence shows that this kind of harm reduction saves lives. If you give heroin to people who are addicted, then they're not prostituting, they're not getting HIV, and they're not killing themselves or others to try to get the resources to obtain heroin. I think it's safe to say that the former Conservative federal government was fairly ideologically driven and not evidence driven on some of their health decisions. That's an example of a socially conservative approach that can actually harm people.

RG: Speaking about delivering health services, you've been the chief health officer for the FNHA in BC for a little less than a year now. How does the FNHA structure work in providing health services?

EA: In Canada, the provinces pay for healthcare services, but status First Nations people are considered federal subjects. There is a separate healthcare system, Health Canada's First Nations and Inuit Health Branch, and they provide services [largely nurse-based] to status First Nations people. In BC, that responsibility has been transferred from the federal government to the FNHA. This means that First Nations people in British Columbia are looking after themselves; Ottawa and their bureaucrats do not look after them.

RG: Are there authorities like this in any other provinces or territories?

EA: There are little tiny authorities: there's one in Manitoba and one in Nunavut, with its tiny population of 40,000. They each have some ability to do this kind of work, but no, we're the first of this kind.

RG: Do you think that a similar system should be applied throughout all provinces and territories?

EA: I do. I do because the federal government running Indigenous health is an extremely patriarchal and inefficient model. The province of British Columbia should be serving all British Columbians, not all British Columbians minus First Nations people. And also, there's a huge amount of bureaucracy. Let's say grandma has a headache on a reserve and she needs Aspirin. To have to apply to Ottawa to get Aspirin is not only bureaucratic, it's expensive because it adds many steps, and it undermines patient independence because they have to apply for care. On top of this, it's also not evidence driven. Instead of a doctor deciding whether grandma gets Aspirin, a clerk in Ottawa decides if grandma gets Aspirin. It's a ridiculous system. It's untenable, unsustainable, expensive, bloated, and it serves the bureaucracy and not the patient.

RG: I want to ask you a bit more about your career and journey to where you are now. When I was young, I always told my mother that I would be a brain surgeon. Now I'm more interested in primary care, especially pediatrics or family medicine, but I've maintained this drive to become a physician throughout my life, even through my liberal arts degree in anthropology. When did you know you wanted to be a physician?

EA: To be very personal, my sister died when I was a little boy. She died quite violently – she was accidentally shot. The chaos around her death very firmly imprinted on my mind that someone should have been there to help me and to help us. All the families, the whole reserve, the police, the ambulance drivers who came to help, the doctors who tried to save her – they all needed to be better organized. That thought, that health services are meant to be efficient and effective, still drives me today. We shouldn't all be standing around not knowing what to do. That girl over there is dying – "Can we get an ambulance here?" "Oh, we can't get an ambulance here." "She has something that I don't understand." Or "She's speaking in a language I don't know." It shouldn't be like that. That's always been with me. Even though I spent some time as an actor telling the stories of Indigenous people, I think I'm in the right place now: trying to achieve a higher level of organization so that all of the people are helped.

■■ **RG:** I remember when I was in intermediate school in rural Alberta, my sister was being bullied for being Aboriginal. I distinctly remember her coming home to my mother crying because somebody had told a joke to her. I distinctly remember this joke, and it was: "What's the difference between an Indian and a picnic table?" And the answer was: "A picnic table can support a family." She was very torn up about this, and I remember questioning why someone would think another person deserved to be talked about in that way.

■■ **EA:** I think we all have our responsibility to tell why we are where we are, because it's your truth. Stories are like evidence – they can point in the direction of the right way to go, and I hope that you don't feel shy to share why you do what you do.

And these stories are hard to tell, aren't they? It makes you feel a bit vulnerable or sad, but it does change people, and I think that kind of honesty can move your classmates and colleagues. I wouldn't shy away

15

from it, although I did shy away from the story of my sister's death for about twenty years because I didn't want to make people uncomfortable.

■■ **RG:** Both my sister and I are in the healthcare field now. Coming back to your becoming a physician, what were the biggest barriers to this?

■■ **EA:** I was distracted. Honestly, I was distracted while I was getting trained. My son was born a couple of months after I started school. Also, I had to work while I was in medical school. I was lucky because I had quite a high-paying job as an actor, but being an actor was distracting. The way I explained it to my dean was it was like being an Olympic athlete – you can't just tell me to stop. I'm doing really well at it and I love it and it's part of my life. And he said, "if you can keep them both, keep them both." So I shot about forty shows while I was in medical school. And it was a killer.

■■ **RG:** I've done some stage acting in local-, university-, and provincial-level theatre. Even at the University of Toronto where I am now, I was in our medical school musical for two years now. I love acting, and I even miss it right now. My question to you: do you miss acting?

■■ **EA:** Yeah, I miss it a lot. I was embarrassed by it for a long time, actually. People said to me, "You could be great – why are you fiddling around with this stupid hobby of yours?" People don't take you seriously when they hear you like to act. It took me a long time to realize that this is what I like to do – it's fun. It's this silly thing I like to do where I stand up and be a fool. Maybe one time I was national level, like being an athlete, but not anymore. That's okay. You can't be good at something forever. It's what makes me happy and it took me forever to get to that confidence.

■■ **RG:** How do you think that your acting career helped you as a physician?

EA: It actually helped me a lot. First, it asked me to be very empathetic, because acting is about empathy and the memory of feelings and situations. I can easily remember being humiliated, being in pain, feeling sad, or needing help. I can remember my patients and how they made me feel, when they lost a baby or when they were maimed forever, and I can connect with them without much effort. And then, as a bit of a celebrity, a lot of Indigenous people know who I am, which meant that they were very friendly with me. They would recognize me and connect with me in a way they wouldn't connect with other doctors.

RG: So you now practise in public health. What do you miss about clinical practice and primary care?

EA: Technically, I'm still in practice, but not clinically, in that I look after populations as opposed to individual patients. But I do miss primary care; I miss listening to moms or taking a medical history. However, my work is similar in that I do subject histories. I'm not dealing with an individual patient, but it's a lot like an individual patient.

RG: Many Indigenous physicians feel as if they're kind of walking between two worlds with western medicine on one hand and Indigenous medicine or teachings on the other. How do you reconcile these two in the work that you do?

EA: I reconcile them in part because I have to. I live with Indigenous people all the time, and they constantly ask me to sing our songs, to dance our dances, and to be with them in ceremonies and in their everyday lives. So I do walk with them. And I do have a traditional medicine godmother who always shakes her head and says, "Such a waste," like I could have been a good healer. But I'm a western doctor, and I constantly remind everyone that I have Indigenous knowledge like many ordinary Aboriginal people, but I am not a traditional knowledge-keeper. Western-trained doctors are great – they're meant to do great things that are helpful, and I'm not a sellout. I just walk those two worlds and I help people cross over between the two.

▪▪ Chapter 2 ▪▪

Being First Nations in Canada: The Rigged Game

Marcia Anderson DeCoteau (Indigenous Physicians Association of
Canada) – Scott Hodgson

*Dr Marcia Anderson DeCoteau currently splits her time working
as an assistant professor within the Department of Community Health
Sciences at the University of Manitoba Faculty of Health Science, as a
general internist at Grace General Hospital in Winnipeg, as a medical
officer of health in northern Manitoba, and as a mother. She graduated
from the University of Manitoba Faculty of Medicine in 2002, completed
her internal medicine residency in Saskatchewan, and completed a Master
of Public Health at Johns Hopkins Bloomberg School of Public Health.
She is past president of the Indigenous Physicians Association of Canada
(IPAC).*

*I first met Dr Anderson DeCoteau at a Canadian Federation of
Medical Students (CFMS) meeting in Winnipeg, in the first month of
medical school in Manitoba. She talked about First Nations, Métis, and
Inuit peoples, and the way that our health system treats them. This talk
would form the basis and drive behind my ongoing interest in Indigenous
health, and my desire to practise family medicine in northern Canada.*

▪▪ **Scott Hodgson:** The social determinants of health are intuitive
to think about, but aren't what a lot of people would think of as a doctor's
work. How do you approach these determinants?

▪▪ **Marcia Anderson DeCoteau:** I think of the social determinants
of health as the policies and legislation that shape social, economic,

19

and environmental factors that contribute positively or negatively to people's health. Healthcare is one of those factors. There is a Canadian Senate report on health that has a diagram estimating that the impact of healthcare is about 20 to 25 per cent of a person's health status. That makes a lot of sense to me. It parallels a quote from David Werner, who is associated with the People's Health Movement: "The health of the people is determined more by politics and economics than by doctors and medicine."

As physicians, we are uniquely situated. We can influence the healthcare system and how we provide care. We can influence the ways we interact with patients and their real lived experience and context, and how to provide the best possible care for them. But we can also use the power that we have as collectives through physician organizations and medical student associations to advocate for better policy and legislation to remove the social injustices that lead to health gaps.

One of the things that the Truth and Reconciliation Commission [TRC] recommended was that as healthcare professionals and systems, we understand that the gaps between First Nations, Métis, and Inuit peoples and the rest of Canada are a direct result of colonization and government policies. The report says past policies but I would say also current. If you read the TRC report, some of the parallels between the underfunding of residential schools and how that negatively impacted health and learning are still things that we see today in the chronic, systematic underfunding of First Nations education systems. From a broad Indigenous community perspective as reflected in the TRC document, the community is asking healthcare providers to see our health as a result of the social determinants of health. We definitely have a responsibility within the healthcare system, but they're also asking us to understand and talk about First Nations, Métis, and Inuit health in the context of colonization.

SH: The social determinants of health definitely apply to all Canadian citizens as a whole, but there's no argument that they have negatively impacted Indigenous communities so much more. There are also a number of factors that only apply to Indigenous communities, such as the residential school intergenerational trauma.

MAD: Displacement from land, not honouring the treaties. Other communities are impacted by racism, too – we do not have a monopoly on racism. But I think that if we were to systematically study it, the depth and frequency of experiences of interpersonal racism would be higher. Also, when we talk about multi-level racism, the institutionalized racism that is embedded in our structures, we have clear legislation about that, right? The Indian Act legally defines you as part of the Indian population or not, and there are Indigenous people who are not recognized, and that can lead to inequities.

SH: Inequities within an already impoverished community; inequalities in a community that is already treated unequally.

MAD: Exactly, and that is a deliberate strategy in and of itself. There a couple of things in that: one is to reduce the federal government's obligation to First Nations people over time by having rules that are designed to "breed out" First Nations by restricting how status can be passed on. It systemically reduces the number of people who qualify. The federal government taking unilateral authority over defining who meets those criteria is against international norms and rights for Indigenous peoples to self-define. The second strategy is to engender competition amongst Indigenous groups. There are some who feel that we are stronger together, but there is real competition for funding for really basic things, like education or access to healthcare or infrastructure. Sometimes at a community level you have to do what's best for your community even if it means competing with those around you. If you're successful, other communities might still be doing poorly.

Even broader than that is setting this national discourse where we as Indigenous people already "get too much." There is no national discourse around what is equitable, what is rights-based, and what is needed in Indigenous health or social spending in order to achieve equitable outcomes. The main discourse is actually "You already get too much," and that's rooted in the other layers of racism and stereotypes about not paying taxes, which is not true for most Indigenous people. But things like not paying taxes and being lazy and unemployed, that is how overlapping discourses and multi-level racism keep status quo structures in place.

SH: Given the historical context, it is actually terrifying how much easier or more common it is currently for Child and Family Services to take a child away from an Indigenous family versus a non-Indigenous family, given the atrocities that the federal government has been involved with in terms of residential schools.

MAD: The policy context has created a health issue or a social issue, but the dominant discourse or tendency is to blame the individual who ends up sick or needing help. You could do the same thing for child welfare. I'm going to use tuberculosis [TB] as an example. There is some debate about whether TB was present in North America prior to European contact. What is certain is that even if it was present, there were not huge epidemics of TB, and that had to do with differences in housing, diet, agriculture, etc. Over time, different policies started to create conditions in which TB could flourish. One was creating these reserve-based systems, in which people had to live in small, confined spaces and were crowded for the first time. Those communities had moved from place to place depending on the season and what they could harvest as hunter-gatherers to feed themselves. That was gone, and now they're in these small, overcrowded spaces. At the same time, there was a complete shift in economy so one could no longer have a hunter-gatherer lifestyle because of the policies around reserves and hunting. And then there was this rations system, which was figuratively and literally white-food based, with things like flour and sugar that we now know are bad for us.

And then traumas started happening. So we have schools that are not built for health. There is a lot of documentation about them not being up to code, lots of fires, and tons of kids being in one little dorm room. You'd never be able to follow proper isolation protocols. So we have TB epidemics in the schools, of course. And that keeps going on until today. There's never been a different policy direction to stop poverty in these designated reserve lands, some of which are on traditional territory and many of which are not. Many of them have had their lands disrupted by mining or hydro or other developments which are of little benefit to the community. So we still see a situation in which a large proportion of First Nations communities have limited economic resources. It is really hard to be healthy if you live in structural poverty. There is a wealth of evidence around that. We also don't have effective food policies, whether you're in the North or in the inner city, and so your access to nutrition is different.

At the same time, with the introduction of the social welfare system post World War II and no opportunities for employment, we saw a real shift to a more sedentary lifestyle. Then layer in trauma and addiction issues that involve food, alcohol, and tobacco, living through the fallout of the residential school experience and the abuses, and housing on reserves that generally would be condemned anywhere else.

Without a doubt, if you look at the state of TB today in Canada, it occurs almost exclusively in Indigenous people. The only other populations that get TB would be immune-compromised people or people who bring it in with them from other countries. So we have created, quite systematically and successfully through policies rooted in either assimilation or decimation, frankly, poor health outcomes. Each system is designed perfectly to get the results that it gets. That was the policy track in Canada, and so it was successful in that it has created ill health, and we've never had a change in that direction. And with TB, as a communicable disease, we've effectively criminalized the person who has basically been funnelled into that position. And I don't want to sound too deterministic, because there are people who are successful in spite of our systems, but that's in spite of and not because of.

Say that your parent or grandparent, thirty or forty years ago in the era of sanatoriums, was removed from their community and you never saw them again. So you're scared to present for treatment or you're scared to take your treatment. You actually could be locked up for being sick as a result of the system that our society created. The advantage of the broader social-determinants perspective is that it allows us to shift our gaze and blaming games from the individual to the system that creates the situation for poor health. The fundamental point of public health is to create the conditions for good health.

■■ **SH:** I recently spent ten weeks working at the nursing station in Split Lake Cree Nation, Manitoba, and much of what we've been talking about definitely relates to my experiences there. Seeing how many people are forced to stay in one house, and then if one person from that house comes in and they have TB, it instantly becomes a huge crisis because now there are ten other people who will most likely get TB. The nurses there were great, they were very caring and everything, but it's just such a built-in part of the medical system that "this person has TB, so we need to force them to take this medicine, and if they don't take this medicine then they're just a terrible person." It's built into the healthcare system to almost instantly criminalize them. ▮▮▮ **MAD:** Well, under the Public Health Act, a diagnosis of TB gives the Province of Manitoba the authority to legislate your actions. That's why it's called TB Control, and they try not to say that as much anymore, but literally they can lock you up and force you to take the pills. And they will.

I don't think there's a very critical discourse about the harms of that. If you're in the system and you identify the one person with TB, and choose to have a public health warrant issued for that person to be locked into a room and take their pills, you can feel some measure of success that you've controlled TB in that person. Once you're no longer infective and you're going for outpatient therapy, you're a lot less likely to get locked up again, as opposed to the initial diagnosis when you're infectious. If people don't complete their treatment, that leads to multidrug-resistant TB, which is a problem worldwide. There is a global public health upside to that kind of enforcement approach. But what happens locally to those ten people, and then the people they're in contact with? One person gets tested and then locked up, how many of those other people are likely to volunteer for testing?

Discrimination in the justice system is a persistent, well-known, nonresolving issue. I have an ethical issue with legislation that almost exclusively targets Indigenous people, and a lot of the Public Health Act is like that. We do need some public health legislation, but we need to be very balanced in the context of our historic and current involvement and the harms of using it.

SH: I believe in patients as storytellers and that there is a lot of good to be had just from listening to somebody's story. And there's a lot of good that comes from being able to tell a story well, especially at my level as a clerk where I need to report that story to a senior doctor. In terms of talking about social determinants of health, do you have any stories that you could share from a personal level that might clarify that concept?

MAD: I had one patient not too long ago referred to me for optimization of his cardiac care. In my practice, I see a lot of cardiology patients as I'm a general internist. On the referral, it actually said he was having difficulty taking his medications because of cost. As a patient with established cardiac disease, you're generally on no less than five medications, and he was diabetic, so he needed a statin [anti-cholesterol medication], Aspirin, Plavix [blood-thinner] for his stents, ACE-inhibitor [anti-hypertensive], beta-blocker [anti-hypertensive], and a couple of diabetes drugs, plus testing strips and a glucometer. Not inexpensive.

Not all Indigenous people have their medications paid for. That's another myth. Non-insured health benefits are for registered First Nations people and some Inuit. He was a non-registered First Nations man, so he did not have access to that. He had more precarious types of employment, as many Indigenous people do. He was still employed but he didn't have benefits in the type of work that he did, so no private insurance. But because he was employed, his deductible for Manitoba Pharmacare was still quite high. And I believe there were some issues with supporting other family members in addition to just him and his wife. Economically, the numbers were just not going to add up. He was in a spot where he could not afford to spend enough on his medications to become eligible for Pharmacare, because it is means-tested based on your income. Instead, he was just choosing which medication to take as he couldn't take them all. In that regard, the key determinant of health was the federal government defining registered First Nations as being the only population that receives non-insured health benefits. Métis and non-registered First Nations have not been eligible for those benefits. Here's an employed, hard-working guy, but he can't afford the medications he needs.

SH: Part-time term positions, or positions that just don't have benefits – that's a structural employment issue. It may be related to education also since education sets you up for what types of employment you can get. It's really tough to be in a room with someone who has worked his whole life and can't afford medications because of the way the system is designed.

MAD: Designed to reduce costs, so that we can have income splitting for people like me, who really don't need those tax cuts because we can afford it. That's a reflection of our societal value collectively and of who votes. Income splitting won't benefit the health of our population at all. It will lead to more income inequality, which we know leads to growing health inequality.

There are two things in the healthcare environment that are important in this case. First, being able to talk to your patients in a way that doesn't make them feel bad about themselves, and putting a focus instead on the systemic failures. You have to show respect for him as a hard-working individual. Second is the importance of referrals. In this case, I did as much as I could to get him through the month, and set him up with a social worker to review his income and look at any other ways that we might be able to facilitate access to medications.

Another story is that of a First Nations woman who lives in Winnipeg, is also diabetic, and has multiple risk factors for heart disease. She presented to hospital with chest discomfort. This is a bit more of a positive story, because I did some tests and decided that she needed an angiogram, and I asked her if she was willing to have it done. She wanted to know what the recovery time would be. And so I was trying to explain that it depends on what they find, and that it could be anything from needing to have nothing done – which is unlikely because of her risk factors – to multi-vessel disease requiring bypass surgery before she gets out of the hospital. For the average person, it would be a couple of days. She said the main reason she was asking was because she's a residential school survivor, and one of the things that she really values as a way to pass on her culture, because she did not get that in the residential schools, is working with young women in the inner city who don't know how to cook traditional foods. That policy choice that led to her going to residential schools interrupted the transmission of knowledge to her about her culture, so she didn't want a medical procedure interrupting her passing on what she knew to the next generation. That's more of a positive social determinants story.

SH: That's a great story. I think that a lot of the time, we tend to focus more on injustice, especially when it comes to Indigenous populations. But I think there are a whole slew of good social determinants that we should be making use of, such as self-determination, traditional knowledge, and healing. In terms of these stories that you encounter all of the time, how do they affect your role as an advocate?

MAD: I see patients half a day a week, and the other 90 per cent of my week is spent almost exclusively in advocacy-type roles. Whether that is through teaching or looking at policy here at the University of Manitoba Faculty of Health Sciences, or in my public health job, the majority of my work is rooted in actions on the social determinants of health.

That was a deliberate decision I made when I was a third- or fourth-year medical student. Even when I did my internal medicine residency, which was kind of hell, I never actually intended on practising clinical medicine full time. I got far too frustrated with the system's inefficiencies and issues. I also thought that even if I was the best doctor ever, if I'm frustrated every day because of systemic issues – not just within the healthcare system, but also the broader-system issues that lead to the majority of patients in internal medicine being Indigenous – then I'm not going to be happy. I'm not going to be fulfilled, and I'm not going to be doing my best. I know that I'm going to have a far broader impact if I set myself up to work at policy-system levels.

SH: Which makes a lot of sense, especially as the metaphor of working upstream rather than downstream is gaining some momentum. Instead of seeing patients after they've already had the problems, you want to be addressing it so that 1) they might not get the problems and 2) if they do get the problems, then it's going to be a much better system for helping them.

MAD: Not only are Indigenous people diagnosed later, but the natural history of the disease and the progression to end-stage complications including kidney failure and lower-limb amputation happens much quicker. That is a result of both inequitable access to care or quality of care, but also because these people have the same living conditions and social environments that contributed to their diabetes, and that situation is going to keep contributing to the poor outcomes from diabetes. So, before the person is in the river, we have the opportunity to keep them out of the river. Once they're in the river, once they've been diagnosed, we have that opportunity to slow their travel down– put them in a boat, keep them above the water, whatever the analogy is.

SH: My current plan is to go into Northern Health for a few years, then switch into public health, as I think it's important to have that first hand-experience, but internal medicine is also interesting. Any advice on this?

MAD: I always thought I would be a pediatrician. Then, in my third year, I went to Zambia for an elective and spent a few months there. That was a great learning experience for me. I felt really useful, and learned a lot. But as I learned more about Indigenous health over the course of medical school, and more about myself as a First Nations woman, I began to realize that this is my passion, and I felt really strongly that my role is to be here and to work with my people at this time.

As far as internal medicine goes, so many of the patients were First Nations, Métis, or Inuit, and the biggest disease burden was from chronic disease. I thought I should set myself up with the best training in chronic disease. That's why I decided to do internal medicine, and then a Master of Public Health.

SH: Speaking about upstream actors and physicians' roles in that, how do you think that we can make physicians more aware of their role in improving social determinants and make it easier for physicians to take action in that regard?

▌▌ MAD: I'm not sure that it is an awareness issue. Some of the actions that would reflect a social-determinants approach are directly counter to what are in the best individual interests of physicians, and sometimes their collective interests as well. Tax benefits, like income splitting, are one of the examples. Realistically, we know that measures that create income inequality benefit the top 20 per cent of income earners, and physicians generally fit into that top 20 per cent.

Part of the question is how you identify the physicians whose values align with an upstream approach. I think the more we talk about it the better, through organizations like Upstream or Canadian Public Health Association or physician organizations. We need to do a much better job defining what advocacy is, and what an appropriate advocacy is. It's in the CanMEDS competencies of what a doctor needs to know, but for the most part it tends to be framed in how you advocate for an individual patient as opposed to how to advocate for populations, and there is generally no strategy around that higher-level advocacy.

The strategy is super important. I'm learning that more and more when trying to build my personal skill set in advocacy. That's something we could do more at a Postgraduate Medical Education [PGME] or Continuing Professional Development [CPD] level, as opposed to a student level where you're just learning the nuts and bolts of medicine. More PGME- and CPD-type education around how to be a better advocate for those who are already on board, rather than trying to convince the ones who aren't on board to get on board, is a better investment. That education should include basic things, like understanding the political process and how policies and legislatures are made, how to get meetings with members of Parliament or members of legislative assemblies, what the federal government regulates versus what the province regulates, and how you reach out and work with other organizations to build those strategic alliances. Those are all really important skills. A lot of us tend to think that if we just write a letter, then they should take our really good advice because we're doctors and that should settle it because that is where the evidence is, but that's not the reality of how policies get made. Until you learn what forms the bedrock of the most effective advocacy, it's really tough and easy to get discouraged when your letters don't go anywhere.

SH: What you're saying is somewhat true of all of medicine. Years three and four will be where I actually solidify what I've learned during the first two years because I'll be practising it every day. Advocacy is the same way: you have to have those nuts and bolts of how does advocacy actually work and then you need to practise it or else you're going to forget.

MAD: And you always build more, right? What you do as a first-year surgery resident is different than what you do as a fifth-year. We need to approach advocacy the same way, in how we teach about it and what we expect of it from the learners.

SH: A previous Canadian Medical Association president said that medical students are the best advocates, just because they're the ones that are out doing that sort of thing. Hopefully we can change that in years to come and bring everybody else up to that level in terms of advocacy.

MAD: There are always tensions around advocacy, too. With the competition for funding, there is always a risk to advocacy. If you're advocating for something that is a position that the government doesn't like, are you shooting yourself in the foot? Medical students are a pretty protected group; there are not a lot of repercussions. That's different than if you're the president of an association that is core funded by the federal government. That's something that can be the scaling-up of learning: how to balance the tensions, how to stay true to your values and advocate without risking your position.

■■ **SH:** There's a famous quotation by Rudolf Virchow that reads, "Politics is medicine on a larger scale." What political changes in Canada do we need to lead to greater health?

■■ **MAD:** Well, one thing that the World Health Organization commission recommended when they did their report on the social determinants of health several years ago now is that each government should assess its performance based on health outcomes, and specifically health equity outcomes. That would be one key thing that we could do at a provincial and federal level.

There's also a whole wealth of evidence that says that the longer and more frequently a country has left-leaning governments, the less income inequality and therefore the less health inequality. So if we want to take a public health, evidence-based approach to elections, then we would all vote for left-leaning parties. Or we could look at those policies that lead to less income inequality, and that lead to less structural racism, but we need to be committed to do that. I know that this is not going to happen, because the number-one consideration in my experience from a policy perspective is "Will we get re-elected in this four-year cycle?" When we're talking upstream, we're talking over generations. So how do we get away from that to think about what is best for the population: health, education, social outcomes? Because those things are all the same. Number-one priority is shifting that discourse. We also need to increase voter turnout, getting people engaged politically, so that we have more democratic influence over policy, and a democracy that is actually more representative of the entire population. We need to be accountable to close the gaps as a performance measure of governance, and we need to look at policies that reduce income inequality and structural racism.

SH: We talked a lot about the inequalities that face Indigenous people, but I think an important concept of that is that in all of the literature I've read, inequality hurts more than just the people who are being held down. Inequality hurts the entire population.

MAD: That's an important point. I mean, there are the moral and ethical reasons that one should care, but really the only way that we're going to make any gains in our population's health as a whole is if we start levelling up those who are bearing the brunt right now.

SH: I mean, if we did that, taxes would go down, expenses for everyone would go down. It's one of those things where it seems so obvious, but it's just so difficult to get buy-in.

MAD: It's so true. But people are constantly anxious, angry, and upset about the proportion of the budget that goes to healthcare spending. So I respond, "Well then, why don't we stop creating conditions of ill health, and start creating conditions of health?" I know it's not that simple, but you at least need to set that direction, right? You need to start by facing upstream.

■■ Chapter 3 ■■

From the Clinic to the Capital: Advocating for Systemic Change

Gary Bloch (Health Providers Against Poverty) – Justin Neves

Dr Gary Bloch is a family physician at St Michael's Hospital in Toronto and an assistant professor in the Department of Family and Community Medicine at the University of Toronto. Dr Bloch has a large clinical practice serving inner-city populations in Toronto, and is the founder and chair of the Ontario College of Family Physicians' Committee on Poverty and Health, a founding member of Health Providers Against Poverty, and a founder of Inner City Health Associates, a group of more than sixty physicians providing primary, mental health, and palliative care in over forty shelters and drop-in centres across Toronto.

There is a fairly recent movement in family medicine encouraging healthcare professionals to prescribe income – a play on the idea that educating patients on their tax returns, for example, can benefit patients' health in the same way counselling on eating healthier or exercising more could. I had the opportunity to chat with Dr Bloch, who was part of the group that coined this term a few years back. We sat down to chat about how he ended up as a leading health advocate in medicine and how the prescribing income campaign fits within a broader understanding of the social determinants of health.

I pursued a career in medicine with the plan that I would use my training as a springboard to engage in all aspects of healthcare – from treating hypertension, to providing resources for social services, to engaging

35

in health policy and systems innovations. Now in my final year of medical school at McMaster University, I often feel worn down and inundated by the amount of new clinical knowledge I am bombarded with every day. Fortunately, mentors like Dr Bloch and the rest of the physicians in this anthology demonstrate to us how we can take advantage of the privilege bestowed upon us to serve our patients and communities in numerous creative ways. Whether you are a trainee or a seasoned physician, I hope you find a story in the following interview that helps you explore new ways to improve health broadly.

▮▮ Justin Neves: How did you get where you are today as a family doctor and strong advocate in the social determinants of health? What were some of the watershed moments for you along this journey?

▮▮ Gary Bloch: That's a big question. To back it up somewhat and trace my path forward, it was pretty clear to me that this was the type of thing I wanted to do, though I didn't know exactly what it would look like. I grew up in a social justice-oriented, Zionist, socialist youth movement. We moved from South Africa when I was young, but I certainly have the story of South Africa very much implanted in my brain as part of my identity. Another part of my identity is the fact that my grandparents had all dealt with being Jewish in a time when being Jewish was difficult. My grandparents escaped Germany in 1939 just before the war.

My undergraduate degree was in African and colonial history, so that gave me some theoretical framework for dealing with social injustice in the world. I didn't know that I would end up in medicine, but it felt like the right place to go after four years in a much more academic context, a chance to marry theory and knowledge with a very practical set of skills. I was definitely nervous going into medicine, about where I would find my new people. When I started medical school at the University of British Columbia, I had to spend a bit of time finding the people to support my vision of what medicine could look like. I think I did find them though. Having Peter Granger, a physician who was very involved in the establishment of a student clinic in the Downtown Eastside, as a mentor was very important for me. He was a very kind, caring, calm, progressive physician who fit into the mainstream of the medical world and helped me bridge those worlds.

JN: So many social issues have an impact on health. Somewhere along the way you took a particular interest in poverty and low-income populations. How did that come about?

GB: I think there are a of couple pieces to that. One – and this is very common to many people who consider themselves progressive or social justice minded – is that you get sucked into an endless number of issues. There is a campaign on everything, and it can become very overwhelming. I have seen people not know how to control that, not know where to pull back, and not know how to focus, and quite honestly not be that effective because they are spreading themselves so thin. So there was certainly a thought in my mind that I would have to focus somewhere, at some point, and couldn't take on the world completely.

My poverty focus happened somewhat by chance. Soon after residency, I got involved in a campaign to raise welfare rates in Ontario. It was led by the Ontario Coalition Against Poverty, a well-known radical anti-poverty group, not one that traditionally allies with doctors at all. They had decided to start up clinics assessing people for something called the Special Diet Allowance, which provided an extra $250 in monthly income, and wanted to find health professionals willing to staff these clinics. I was part of a small initial group of providers who got involved.

What was amazing about that campaign for us was that as we looked at regulations around the Special Diet program, we realized that they were very loose. We decided that we could legitimately prescribe every person in these clinics who lived on welfare the full $250 per month supplement based on the diagnosis of poverty, given the health evidence that we have linking poverty with poor health outcomes. This was a real eye-opener for me. It suddenly gave us a whole new role within anti-poverty social justice movements. This was very much a campaign led by people affected by poverty and living with low income. Suddenly, we were able to directly intervene, to essentially use medical skills to address poverty. Prescribing income was the catchphrase that came out of that work.

Income is quite honestly a catch-all social determinant of health. Low income is common ground for those who experience the most vulnerability and marginalization, and can help us build a more complex analysis of what that means. The other piece is that poverty is something very easy for people to understand. So as opposed to coming in talking about the intersectionality of multiple social issues, we are talking about people living without enough money to survive, or at least to afford to live the kind of lives they deserve to live.

The other lesson that came for me out of the Special Diet campaign was that if we wanted to expand this beyond this initial group of about eighty health providers in that campaign, we would have to be a little smarter about how we messaged and marketed this idea. The subsequent ten years of work have really largely been about that – about repackaging this idea to bring the much broader health world on board.

JN: There are so many opportunities for doctors, especially family doctors, to engage in this kind of work, not just treating patients' hypertension and diabetes with medication, but looking at what they are eating and why they are eating that way – tracing these factors upstream. How do we continue to push the envelope and engage more physicians in these kinds of discussions and programs?

■■ **GB:** I use two catchphrases here. One of them is using the stages-of-change approach, which is obviously borrowed from the addictions literature, which is the idea that you have to meet people where they are and push them incrementally. So if there are doctors who have never thought about intervening in a social issue in their career, you can't then expect them to jump out to the front lines of a protest or write a policy paper. But if you can help them start screening patients for low income to find out who in their practice lives in poverty, hopefully that will evolve into them wanting to do something about it.

The other catchphrase I tend to use is a trickle-up approach, the idea being that successful experiences with basic interventions will trickle up into higher order ones, and wanting to deal with the more systemic issues. One of the basic interventions we offer health professionals is a clinical tool on poverty, which is basically a four-page handout but looks like a clinical tool on diabetes or heart disease. This tool lays out a very simple three-step approach to poverty that can be used by primary-care providers in front-line offices in ten- to fifteen-minute appointments: screening everyone, taking into account the evidence linking poverty and poor health, and very basic interventions to increase income directly through available social programs. This is the sort of stuff that should be very easily incorporated into front-line practice.

■■ **JN:** That's true. I think more and more people are getting on board with the idea that it's part of the physician's role to understand the social context behind people's health. There is the individual branch where the physician is working one-on-one with patients, and there is the population-level branch where we are looking more at health policies and systems-level thinking. What do you think the role is for physicians working in that population-level branch?

GB: Physicians have a long history of involving themselves in public-policy discussions, so I don't think it is new to suggest that physicians should get themselves involved in thinking about higher-level systemic issues, which is certainly what I would advocate. The physician world has realized for a very long time that it is hard to deal with most health issues without thinking about the systemic factors that influence those issues. Whether that is obesity, smoking, heart disease, food, all these things interlink with each other. These are the kinds of issues that the medical world had been very willing to engage with at a very high level, including media campaigns, deputations to governments, attempts to influence policy, and attempts to influence legislation that have an impact on population health in a very broad way.

Many of us are very aware of the fact that some of the greatest advances in health have come from population and public health interventions like sanitation, vaccinations, etc., and not through the front-line, nitty-gritty interventions that physicians spend most of our time doing. We really cannot improve health without dealing with the factors that cause people to have health problems on a systemic basis.

JN: In 2014, the Harper government limited the role of the chief public health officer of Canada to an advisory role on strictly public-health matters, and appointed a president to manage budget and staffing of the Public Health Agency of Canada. Articles and opinions have been published suggesting that the role of physicians working in public health should be focused on disease surveillance and infection rates. So there is still that perception out there. What would you say to those people to try to change that attitude?

GB: I think that those types of comments are very politically driven. There is this idea amongst a certain part of the political spectrum that it is dangerous to have health professionals delving into social issues, because when we do, we tend to push a more progressive view. If you look at the health evidence, it really points us toward a more interventionist role for government in social issues that involves real attempts to level the playing field. This speaks very much against the austerity-driven, right-wing ideologies that have tended to dominate politics lately. It doesn't surprise me that those attempts have been made. We are lucky, though, that we can fall back on the evidence. Another piece of our program has been to always remain as evidence-focused as possible. It is very hard to argue against strong evidence that has been proven over and over again, from many different angles, in many different settings, by many different people, and consistently shows the same thing, which is that these specific social factors influence health.

JN: I am someone whose true passion probably lies with the higher-level policy and program interventions, and this was the type of work I was engaging in before applying to medicine. Through that, I have been exposed to health advocacy from the non-physician perspective (academics, other healthcare workers) as well as the physician/medical-student perspective. How effective do you think physicians are at working together with other stakeholder groups at this systems level? There have been some critiques of medical professionals that they may not give the same respect or the same voice to other stakeholders trying to engage in this work.

GB: I think many of us are very conscious that we work with people who have too often been marginalized and had their voices pushed aside. We very consciously want to find ways to counteract that. There's a flip side to this too, which is that the physician voice is listened to. There's a fine line between wanting to make positive use of the privilege and power that comes with the position, but also not further marginalizing the people that we are ostensibly trying to help.

So what are some answers to that? I don't know that I have absolute answers, but my experience is that it's important to get involved in campaigns that are being designed and led by the people most affected by the issues that are being talked about. Secondly, we need to be very conscious of what our realm of influence and expertise is. So when I come into this work, I try as much as possible to stay within the bounds of what the health evidence tells me and offer up that perspective as a health professional. With that, I bring stories that I deal with as a physician on the front lines, but still offer these up humbly and with the acknowledgement that it's not my story. Finally, I try as much as possible to work physically side by side with the people most affected by these issues.

JN: I particularly liked the point about working from the realm you know best. I think it can be detrimental when the person with the MD after their name starts making statements across multiple disciplines without supporting health evidence. I think we run the risk at that point of clouding the message of other stakeholders that may have more experience and knowledge on a particular subject or issue.

GB: I can tell you that this morning I was at Queen's Park [Ontario's provincial legislative assembly] talking about changes to the Employment Standards Act, talking about basic rules around decent work in Ontario. The piece that I was offering up was one around the social determinants of health and how they relate to sick-pay provisions and disability issues – very clearly pieces that fall within my expertise. I was certainly not stepping in trying to claim that I understand the entire employment standards world. You know the retired judge and high-profile retired partner of a big law firm would never buy that. These guys are sitting there running the commission, so you have to be very conscious of what you are bringing to the table.

■■ **JN:** A few years back there was the "Code Red" series done by the Hamilton Spectator looking at the different neighbourhoods within Hamilton and how they stacked up on different health indicators. It reported that there is a twenty-one year difference in life expectancy between Hamilton's best and worst neighbourhoods, thirteen times difference in the rate of emergency room visits, and ninety times difference in high school dropouts. How does it make you feel when you hear these statistics, showing the kind of inequality of health outcomes in downtown cities like Hamilton or where you work in Toronto?

■■ **GB:** You know this is the reality that we deal with every day. "Code Red" did a very good job of bringing this home for Canadians to show them what was happening right in front of their eyes. Those numbers are astounding, right, when you see them laid out that way and see that neighbours have this difference in life expectancy that we can boil down to social environments. I would hope that that has filtered up to change the way that Hamilton conducts its business, and I would also hope it affects how Ontario conducts its business, and then I certainly have this hope that it has an effect on how health professionals conduct their business. I think the statistics are probably the same for Toronto, but Hamilton was lucky to have a newspaper to sponsor this type of analysis and then spread it really far and wide.

■■ **JN:** Being fortunate to have this opportunity one-on-one,

I wanted to ask you a few more personal questions. Something I struggle with is starting to engage with patients about the issues they are facing. It is easy for me as a twenty-five-year-old to identify with the other twenty-five-year-old that presents to the ER because he injured his shoulder playing football or soccer. It is much harder for me to empathize and understand where someone is coming from who's been homeless for the last two years, who doesn't have a support system, or who doesn't know where their next meal is coming from. Is this something you have ever struggled with, and what would you say to learners who have also struggled with these same things?

■■ **GB:** I think we all struggle with this. It is well known that people applying to medicine typically come from the higher socio-economic strata of society; so we have some barriers to leap in order to truly understand the experience of people who come from lower socio-economic strata. It's helpful to always be conscious of those differences, to be aware and open about where you have come from, what your background is, what sort of privileges you've been able to take advantage of to get where you are. Even if you didn't come from privilege, consider the privilege you enjoy now, because even those coming from more disadvantaged backgrounds have leapt way up the social-class hierarchy the second they step into medical school. We all know how banks love to fawn over medical students. So one piece is the awareness and self-analysis, and the other piece is a real willingness to hear stories – to sit back and to listen to what patients' experiences are and to always assume we do not know what is happening to the patient, what they have been through, and what has led them to where they are when they're sitting in front of you. Let them lay that out by actually giving them space to tell their story.

Everyone has a story. Usually when you are feeling frustrated about someone's health situation or someone's inability to follow our directives about their health, there is almost always a very good reason for that. They may not be able to make that link exactly or immediately, and we certainly won't right away, but through exploring stories it comes out. Sometimes it takes years to find out that history of trauma, for instance, which sort of creates an "aha moment" and you say, "Okay, now I understand why your life feels so chaotic and disorganized. You can't do anything I recommend you do, but I get it. You have this massive wall sitting between you and your ability to improve your well-being, so now we can start chipping away at that wall." But without listening, you will never even see the wall. It will stay invisible, but it is very much physically there. We teach this all the time. We teach this to medical students, residents, practising physicians, that the first step is always to sit back and hear stories and to properly understand a full sense of someone's social situation, their life situation, their life story.

▮▮ **JN:** What has been a particularly rewarding experience that you have had where a patient's story has really come full circle, a moment where you have said to yourself, "This is why I do what I do."

▮▮ **GB:** I'm thinking of a patient I saw today. I do a lot of work in homeless shelters. I have worked in homeless shelters since I started my career. I met this guy two years ago now in the shelter. He was a guy who literally has been living outside nonstop for twenty-five years in a tent, part of it out West and then in Toronto through winter, through summer, not in shelters, never housed, had no contact with any social supports, family, friends, nothing. He was completely alone. He had suffered through a series of heart attacks out in the bush where he literally had to crawl out of the forest onto the highway. He tells the story of trying to wave a car down to take him to the hospital but no one would stop because he looked so dishevelled, so he had to walk into town in the middle of a heart attack to go to the hospital.

He eventually ended up in my clinic in a homeless shelter, and luckily with a case manager in the program that I work with. We started to talk to him about his health and his past and it turned out that he'd finally decided that maybe this was not the most comfortable lifestyle, maybe there could be a way for him to get out of the bush and into housing, but he had no idea what that meant at that point. He agreed to stick with our plan of getting an apartment and bringing him in and starting to work on his health issues, starting to just reconnect him with life. Over the last six to eight months or so, he has reconnected with his sister, which was a huge moment for him, and eventually reconnected with his father as well, and dealt with some issues there. He had not seen his family in over twenty-five years. He just came into my office after cataract surgery and he was literally jumping around the office talking at the top of his lungs about the fact that he could see again. He said he had never noticed that he had grey hair until he came out of the surgery and looked in the mirror. This is how bad his eyesight was, and what he was dealing with. He shook my hand over and over and over and over again, he was so excited.

There is a lot of history here in terms of the traumas and experiences he has been through, but the fact that he sees our part in his path to recovery as being so huge and so significant to him is incredibly satisfying. Every time he comes in he is astoundingly grateful, which is quite amazing to see. I wish I had seen him in the bush for a point of comparison, but I can only imagine what he was like back then. I know what he is like when he comes into my office. He wasn't a very easy guy to connect with, but it didn't take very long to break through that veneer.

■■ Chapter 4 ■■

Shared Decision-Making: An Alternative to Physician-Centred Care

Vanessa Brcic (Basics for Health) – Irfan Kherani

Dr Vanessa Brcic is a family physician and clinical scholar in the Department of Family Practice at the University of British Columbia. She graduated from McMaster University with an interdisciplinary honours degree in arts and science in 2001, and subsequently with her medical degree in 2006.

I felt privileged to have had the opportunity to meet with Dr Brcic in a quaint coffee house in Yaletown, Vancouver. Our common interest in the intersection of medical education and social advocacy set the basis for a conversation on the service we must all provide to underserved populations. Through conversations on her work and approach to medicine, I developed a greater appreciation for the vastness of her experience as a physician, as an advocate, as a citizen, and probably most interestingly, as a person.

Dr Brcic focuses her clinical time in the interdisciplinary care of vulnerable patients and those with complex chronic conditions. Our conversation impressed upon me a realization that primary health is, in and of itself, a form of grassroots-level medical advocacy, especially in underserved populations. Her experiences in rural mental health, addictions, and elder care illustrate how each and every physician can take ownership of ensuring that all populations have access to high-quality care.

We had the opportunity to chat about some personal experiences, including her interests in the outdoors and homesteading activities, and how these experiences have impacted her professional life. We explored how a bicycle-motor vehicle collision in 2010 provided her first-hand experience of the troubles of navigating the healthcare system as a patient. To this end, she now dedicates most of her clinical work to chronic pain.

Dr Brcic co-founded Basics for Health Society in 2014, a non-profit organization aimed at helping patients connect with resources in the community through mentorship with health sciences students. She currently serves as research associate with the BC office of the Canadian Centre for Policy Alternatives, vice-chair of communications for Canadian Doctors for Medicare, and as a partner with the BC Health Coalition and the Public Health Association of BC.

■■ **Irfan Kherani:** Tell me a bit about yourself. What are your interests? Why do you get involved in social advocacy?

■■ **Vanessa Brcic:** Something had been bothering me since I was a medical student: I noticed that, especially in clinical environments, there is always more demand for doctors' services than there is supply. There is always a line-up of people waiting for services, and those people who come knocking are usually people with the best access – the most privileged. It's actually those who don't come knocking who generally need our help the most. Unfortunately, our system is not set up to deal with the people we aren't seeing; our system is set up to deal only with those we are.

There is so much need. And because of that, we are doing less preventative work and focusing on downstream symptom management. As a result, we are creating an illness-care system. Social or environmental issues largely determine which people will suffer most from illnesses.

As a resident, I had a patient who came into our downtown

48

Vancouver clinic – generally a pretty wealthy population, but people travel all over to see a doctor they like. This woman, I would never have guessed, was low-income. She came in one day with her five-year-old drinking a Red Bull. I was immediately alerted that there was something going on in her life, so I just asked a few more questions. The patient had recently been through a divorce and was having some financial troubles, complicated by significant conflict with her partner. I would never have guessed it by seeing her: she was well dressed, she had a cell phone. At that point in time, I became aware that we needed to start screening for poverty, just like we screen for cancer and other diseases. We take a social history, but we rarely incorporate it into the medical history. Reading case reports in journals, I am amazed by the lack of social context.

Before I went into medicine, I worked in community development for a non-profit for a couple of years through the Canadian International Development Agency (CIDA), both inside and outside of Canada. While my main work was a rescue project for kids, it was actually very much a community health development project. The team saw a need in a community for kids to have a transition house after being removed from their home environments. They arranged interventions with affected families to see if the children could go back to their initial homes or if they needed to be housed elsewhere. Once the kids were living in the transition home, they were given access to physical and mental health services. In essence, they collected the most vulnerable kids, those most at risk of exposure to violence, and ended up giving them healthcare.

While I was interested in public, population, and community health, I started to see primary care as grassroots community health development. If primary care is situated in a community, then we can use clinical experiences to understand broader health issues and risks in the community. That is why I was so committed to working on poverty and social determinant issues. It just seemed so much at the core of what we do in primary care.

IK: As we look for options for learners to engage in social advocacy and poverty alleviation, even just choosing primary care is a method.

VB: Certainly. I also think interdisciplinary teams are key. Physicians often fall into a niche of prescribing. While we try to deliver compassionate care complete with counselling, other health professions including nursing, occupational therapy, and counselling have a much more integrated use of social determinants in their patient workup. The more team-based care you can deliver, the more you end up talking about the social determinants. Some of my most rewarding experiences were working as a resident on a mental health interdisciplinary team in Vancouver.

Practising on a long-term care team, you get to appreciate the family story. The patient may not be disclosing how satisfied or happy they are, but through a team, you can start to see the broader picture, which makes the care so much more rewarding. It makes it so much easier when you get a call when you know the patient's story. You know how much you need to worry. Working in care teams really allows me to actively incorporate social determinants into my practice.

IK: One thing you touched upon before was recognizing poverty in the populations that we serve and gave an interesting case that you saw as a resident. We check blood pressure and screen for other conditions; are poverty-screening tools the types of things we should be integrating into our daily practice?

■■ **VB:** For sure. It helps to establish a risk profile of your patients. We use electronic medical records to gather and check in with patients who are at increased risk; the idea that we could identify if there are risks about a person's low income or poverty would be incredible. But you have to be careful when you screen for poverty. You don't want to start talking about it and just add more burdens onto a person's plate. For example, I struggle to pay my rent at the end of the month, I struggle to afford childcare, and now I am at risk of diabetes, and now I have to start eating healthier as well. We have to be careful to not just biomedicalize everything, turning poverty into another medical risk factor that patients have to worry about.

■■ **IK:** How do you find that balance?

■■ **VB:** You have to create a relevant action plan for patients. It's important to recognize that poverty is a risk factor, but that as a wealthy privileged person, placing that label on someone can be detrimental. But if you create an action plan out of it, you can use it as an opportunity to build more patient-centred care and shared decision-making. I see it as building a team between the patient and me. I know more about their life circumstances; I am better able to offer them advice. I am better able to say, "Maybe our action plan this week is going to be helping you find someone to help you with your tax returns. You don't really need that blood work right now, but let's get you filling out some forms."

■■ **IK:** Are we preparing our learners? If you had asked me to do that kind of a comprehensive assessment of a patient, I am not sure I would feel comfortable having that conversation right now as a junior resident. Is there anything that we can do better to prepare students to have those conversations?

■■ VB: I think part of it is framing. If you can take a sexual history, you can take a poverty history. There are a lot of things that are uncomfortable in medicine. You need to come from a place of openness, compassion, and nonjudgment; you also need the tools.

We have founded a not-for-profit organization called Basics for Health Society. It's based on HealthLeads USA, which is a model that has been going on for more than ten years in the United States. It trains students, future healthcare providers, as patient-resource navigators to connect patients to appropriate patient community resources to meet needs related to social determinants of health. The doctor can have a prescription pad where they tick off certain issues, and the patient takes that to the volunteer, and that person tries to find resources in the community. This person will then connect you to community resources and will track what your needs are and get back to your GP.

■■ IK: It closes the loop.

■■ VB: Yes, but it is also an educational experience. Our idea is to expose students to a broader view of health that includes the social determinants. There is a range of students from different health disciplines who want to see how the health and social services system works here.

The program is challenging because of the gaps in community services. Housing is a huge concern. BC Housing in British Columbia is very problematic. The wait-lists are long. There is very little we can do about people's housing concerns. We ask the volunteers, given how hard it is to feel how much people are struggling and given how many gaps there are in the system, "why do you want to do this? Why do you want to even do this as a volunteer? You aren't even getting paid." The volunteers respond by saying that the program opens their minds to the person's story. They feel that they are actually providing a service. Sometimes, the act of being there as a witness for the person's challenges is enough to help that person feel not marginalized, not excluded. People often feel that these issues of food and housing don't belong anywhere. Through the program, we make people feel that we aren't looking away, that we are validating their challenges. As part of our project, we are tracking the gaps in the system. When we aren't able to connect people to resources, is it because it's hard to identify the needs, or is it hard to find the resources because the resources just don't exist?

When the resources are lacking, then we can scale that up to advocate at the population or policy level. The project is creating capacity and actually doing the work of connecting people to resources to address issues around income and social determinants.

▮▮ **IK:** You have written about the "complex paths to healing." This made me think about the multiple variables that are involved in the healing process.

▮▮ **VB:** When people have a lot of barriers to overcome, they often have fewer resources with which to address them. It creates this cycle of marginalization. When you add stigma into that, it becomes even harder. Healing is very much to do with belonging: feeling that you are not an outlier, feeling that you are looked after. A patient never wants to hear that they are an interesting case. They want to be the run-of-the-mill case. When I think of healing, I think of belonging, of reassurance. When someone has a lot of barriers, it's much more complex to envision all of the supports that they need.

▮▮ **IK:** Have you had any specific experiences or stories that you have encountered as a physician or even just as a person that have increased your appreciation for the environment within which we live? Any personal experiences that you draw on to give you the drive to push further?

█▌ **VB:** I was involved in a really bad accident five years ago. I was hit by a car while riding my bicycle and have struggled with chronic pain since then. The program that runs Basics for Health is actually funded by Pain BC, a provincial pain advocacy organization. I also work in a pain clinic. I have had a lot of experience in the pain realm, on the research side and on the clinical side as well as as a patient. I am starting to see that pain is not altogether different from other complex medical issues or issues of barriers with respect to social determinants.

Medicine is focused on individual systems and algorithms to address specific problems. But when there is a global issue incorporating multiple realms of a person's existence, it becomes harder to address. Medicine tends to not want to open that big black box. We are already strapped for time and for resources. If we open the door to talking about a person's social issues, where do you stop? One of the participants in my focus group said, "I am afraid to open that door because I have a whole waiting room of patients waiting for me. What will happen to me if I open that door for that specific patient and everyone else is waiting? Do I have to do the same for everyone else? Is it ethical to ask and then say that we don't have enough time to talk about it today?"

I have seen that play out with chronic pain. How people live with chronic pain is just as complex as opening the door to social determinants. It's an issue that physicians often ask, "Do we really want to open the door to this issue?" One in five people in Canada live with chronic pain, and yet we don't have nearly enough services for those people. We treat the orthopedic issue, we treat the rheumatologic issue, but what about how the person's symptoms affect the day-to-day experience?

I have practised in addictions medicine in the past, and because of my personal experience, have moved more into the pain side of things. I find the most fascinating parts of medicine are the complex ones. When you can situate someone's clinical presentation in the context of their story, it becomes so much more fascinating. Really partnering with the person and bearing witness to their whole story has a huge healing impact. A lot of what I do at the pain clinic is validating people's symptoms. It's often, "We don't have an explanation for your pain, therefore it must not exist." Similarly with poverty, because there is nothing we can do about it, we are not going to ask about it. Overcoming those labels and digging deep and bearing witness to the person's experience are incredibly important.

IK: At the beginning, we chatted about your interests and that the reason why you got involved stemmed from an appreciation for a scarcity of resources. Now, we are talking about how to really get to the core of someone's challenges. How do you reconcile those against each other? What do we tell the physician who has a hundred patients waiting for him?

VB: All of this boils down to the principles of patient-centred care and shared decision-making. You have to be on the same team as the patient. You have to understand what you think is a priority for them and see if it matches what they think is a priority for them. If we can understand each other in that way, then I think it is a successful visit.

We have to be careful about physician-centric care. We do not know what the person is coming in for. Sometimes, the patient experience is focused on symptoms and they don't want to worry about screening for colon cancer. Maybe they have had a haemorrhoid in the past, and they don't really care if it is colon cancer, they just want to get rid of the bleeding because it bothers them. It is your job to inform them of the risks and get them on the team for prevention.

There are certain circumstances where you have to take a stronger stance. Once I had a patient who came in, who was a young guy, and his knee was swollen. His whole leg was swollen with phlebitis, and it was obviously a septic joint and he had let it go. He had had a cut, and it had turned into this chronic issue. He was refusing to go into the emergency department. He came in with his mom, and I physically blocked the door. It's rare that I actually stand up to patients in that way, but I told him that his entire leg was at risk. I told him that I appreciated his issues with the medical profession and his dislike for taking prescription drugs, and the fact he would be waiting at the emergency department for hours. Those were all true, but I told him that he was risking his limb.

There are very few situations that I have to stand up to patients in that way. For the most part, you hear what is going on with them, and you kind of add your knowledge to it, and through that you come to a place of agreement. That's what shared-decision, informed-consent, and patient-centred care is all about. Those are important principles for the practice of good medicine that are present in every discipline. When you lend a social determinants lens to all of those important tools, it makes sense.

■■ **IK:** Thinking upstream is a helpful metaphor – instead of only standing downstream trying to help all those drowning in a river, why not head upstream to find out why people are falling in, to help solve problems at their source? We talked about how this was part of the reason why you jumped into medicine in the first place. What would you say to physicians who are uncomfortable about having those upstream conversations?

VB: As physicians, we don't want to miss anything. We want to make sure that we are being comprehensive about medical care. But sometimes we can get so involved in the minutia and in the downstream issues that we forget to lift our heads above water. Doing so requires us to step back from the clinical symptoms, back from the patient coming in with ten or twelve issues.

I have done a lot of research and work on advocacy, and amongst all the CanMEDS roles, advocacy is the least understood. Doctors can see advocacy as getting their patient an MRI faster. That's an important element, but I think that we are not used to seeing the upstream issues. We are so busy with the downstream effects that it takes a while to separate ourselves.

So long as we are so busy with the downstream issues, we are trapped. Thinking outside of the box, thinking creatively, is really inspiring. I think students are so overwhelmed by understanding the renal system, for example – there is so much that you want to know so as to ensure that you are making good recommendations to patients, that it's hard to step back. If students demanded that space to think more broadly of their schools, I think residency programs would respond quite well. Schools have a tough time teaching advocacy. They don't know how to teach meaningfully about social determinants. With Basics for Health, we are providing one experience for people on how to actually appreciate the social determinants. So if students stand up and say that the social determinants are an important part of our work, and that we all come into medicine with dreams about the society that we want to build, we can optimize the experiences we give our learners.

There are huge community movements for local foods, for active transportation, for a greener economy, and for more sustainable cities. These movements are happening all around us, and they are related to health, but we don't have the time for it. We know that cynicism increases as you go through medical school, as you get sucked into this machine of the biomedical focus. As such, students are important in bringing about this change and focus to medical schools.

■■ **IK:** I agree completely. My initial interest in social advocacy and community engagement was through an education standpoint. I think students and residents are developing a greater sense of where our role as physicians sits within the realm of multidisciplinary teams for community development. Looking at your practice, if you were talking to yourself fifteen years ago, what would you tell yourself?

■■ **VB:** I have always been interested in social determinants, so I had to choose between going into public health or clinical work. When I was actively deciding between them, I remember my dad saying, "You are working in the non-profit sector already; if you go into public health, they'll probably spit you out to work in the same area. You will go to school; you will be inspired by ideas. You will think more about community health, social determinants, community engagement, and development. It will be a really nourishing environment. But if you go into medicine, it won't be nourishing those interests, but we need more of that in medicine. It's going to be more of a battle, but it will spit you out in a different discipline that needs that change to happen." So he asked me, "Which one do you need more in your life? Do you need a nourishing academic environment where you can really grow the interests you already have, or do you have the capacity to take a different path to fight for social justice and social determinants that is not as obvious? It's not the mainstream."

I ended up choosing medicine, for a lot of reasons. It definitely feels like an uphill battle, and I definitely feel like the minority. In medical school, they basically left out community health. I was going through this intense experience of medical school with basically no exposure to my area of interest, which was really hard. So what I would say to myself fifteen years ago is, stick it out. If you have perspectives that aren't shared by your discipline, it's just a way to encourage more thought and more ideas. We need to encourage dialogue about what the profession can do. As much as medicine has its own culture, which is somewhat isolated and pretty individualistic, physicians are part of a broader community. You need to see yourself as part of something bigger.

Remember what really drives you, what really makes you excited. Don't just get caught up in guidelines and differential diagnoses. Try to keep thinking broadly and creatively about a person's health. Creativity and innovation are what keep us all excited. What gives people satisfaction in their work is a sense of ability to enact change, and a sense of empowerment and control over their work. In medicine, we sometimes feel that we are cogs in a machine, drowning in downstream health issues. If we can divert a little bit of energy to think innovatively and a bit upstream, it can be really motivating.

■■ **IK:** That magnifying aspect of it, if you invest just a bit of time in the upstream factors, it can have huge impacts.

■■ **VB:** That's what motivates me, and what allows me to work with such complex patients: addictions, chronic pain, elderly patients with mental illness. These aren't easy populations to work with, but I have found them quite rewarding. They allow me to look at these complex cases at a community level and say, "Hmm, what can we be doing systematically to improve the situation?" I am doing something systematically, so I am not so discouraged when I see someone with so many barriers because I know I am also working upstream to try to address them.

▪▪ Chapter 5 ▪▪

What's a Life Worth?

Naheed Dosani (Palliative Education and Care for the Homeless) –
Jesse Kancir

Being sick, of course, is very hard, but being sick and living on the street is even harder. Dr Naheed Dosani is a passionate and respected advocate for marginalized and vulnerable populations with palliative needs. He serves as a palliative care physician at Inner City Health Associates and William Osler Health System in Brampton, Ontario. After completing his family medicine and palliative care training, Dr Dosani founded Palliative Education and Care for the Homeless (PEACH). Through PEACH, he provides Toronto's most marginalized populations with compassionate care and a dignified approach to their end-of-life journeys.

Prior to interviewing Dr Naheed, I knew of him because of his social media presence. He actively engages in public discussions involving health and in my mind is one of the most publicly engaged new-in-practice physicians. During our interview, I appreciated his passion and empathy. For Dr Naheed, concern for his patients' health is not simply an occupation or an academic pursuit. This is about being a neighbour and a citizen of a community.

▪▪ **Jesse Kancir:** What drew you to medicine as a profession, and more specifically, to family medicine and palliative care?

▪▪ **Naheed Dosani:** I think a lot of the inspiration to be in medicine was to work in a field where I may be able to enable and empower social change. My parents are from a small country in East Africa called Uganda and in the early 1970s, dictator Idi Amin came to power. His policies were very discriminatory and he actually ethnically cleansed the country. And so my parents came to Canada as refugees in 1972. You know how there is a lot of talk about the Syrian refugees right now? Well in 1972 it was the Ugandan Asian refugee crisis. And so I was raised by parents who had lived the refugee experience, and I heard about their various struggles. What my parents went through was always an interest for me. Certain messages really resonated for me, like the idea to obtain an education and utilize that education to make a difference in the life of others. Now, engineering and law obviously came to mind, but medicine started to make sense to me when I started to read the trials and tribulations of people like Richard Heinzl or James Orbinski of Médecins Sans Frontières. I started to realize that through medicine we have the opportunity, from the individual to the population perspective, to empower social change, and that really inspired me.

When I was thinking about various specialties, the goal was to try and find one that allowed me to focus on change. Since the beginning, it felt innate in family medicine to advocate for social change. In family medicine, we have the opportunity to link patients to a whole host of supports, to truly represent their voices. Further, we are a resource to our patient population and have the opportunity to advocate both individually and from a population perspective. When I completed my residency at St. Michael's Hospital at the University of Toronto, I became very aware of how the social determinants of health could be integrated into a primary care model. It made a lot of sense that one could be enabled to empower social change through the social determinants.

When I started to do my family medicine residency, we did an inner-city block, working in the shelter system where we had to work to support patients with serious diseases. One case really impacted me: a gentleman in his late thirties who presented to the infirmary floor of the shelter with a pain crisis. As I got to know him and learn more about his background, I realized that he had been marginalized for a lot of his life. He had a history of mental illness (he had been diagnosed with schizophrenia), and he knew he had cancer. But all he was seeking was the kind of analgesic pain control that you and I would so easily get if we had the need for that type of care. He went from emergency room to emergency room, walk-in clinic to walk-in clinic, hospital to hospital, seeking comfort.

When I returned to the shelter one day, I couldn't find him in his dorm or in the cafeteria. So I asked one of his roommates what had happened to him. His roommate said that he had died overnight. He had come rushing into the room in the middle of night, saying he was in pain and that no one cared for him; he said he wanted to die. He went out onto the street and, sadly, died on a combination of opiates, alcohol, and benzodiazepines.

That story is a sample size of one. But it really became the impetus to investigate what the social determinants experience was like for those who are marginalized and vulnerable and experiencing a life-limiting illness.

I actually had to take some time off because this story hurt me so dramatically, so emotionally that I needed to really reflect upon what I wanted to do. During that time, I started to understand the plight of the population. I found that there were thirty-six publications in the literature about the plight of people who are homeless and who have life-limiting conditions and what the quality of their life is like. And I learned some things that really shocked me: that the life expectancy of a homeless person in a metropolitan area like Toronto or Vancouver is thirty-four to forty-seven years old. The mortality rates are 2.3 to 4 times higher than the Canadian baseline population.

Did you know that 90 per cent of Canadians want to die at home, as per the Canadian Hospice Palliative Care Association? I learned that among the homeless, 35 to 60 per cent of this population dies in acute care settings when they actually just want to die at home like many Canadians do. And it got me thinking that in palliative care, you have the opportunity to support every patient who can benefit from a palliative approach, especially the vulnerable. Because in our healthcare system, patients with life-limiting illnesses are vulnerable, and when you layer on the diseases of the social determinants of health, such as homelessness or poverty, you have an extra layer of vulnerability that is truly shocking.

What you end up with is a subset of the population that struggles day-to-day due to food insecurity, homelessness, and poverty. As they approach the end of life, their journey is marred by premature death and often lacks the dignity that all people truly deserve. So for me, the decision to practise palliative care for marginalized populations was a logical choice. This is why I worked with colleagues at Inner City Health Associates in Toronto to establish and found a new model of care, called Palliative Education and Care for the Homeless (PEACH). PEACH is a mobile, street- and shelter-based supportive and palliative care service for Toronto's homeless and vulnerably housed population with serious and/or life-limiting illnesses.

■■ **JK:** You have this very rich personal history with a family that immigrated to Canada. You brought that in right away and talked about vulnerability and applied that to marginalized populations. Would you say that understanding of vulnerability has been a constant attraction to you throughout your life or as you have gone through undergrad medicine, family medicine, and palliative care training? Has dealing with different populations given you a different perspective on medicine?

■■ ND: I think that progression throughout medical training has shown me the basic tenets of medicine: acute medicine, preventive medicine – you know, all of the specialties you rotate through and how they're so important to patient care. But in each of those rotations, in each of those units in the pre-clerkship curriculum, is a layer of the social determinants that I think more and more medical schools are trying to incorporate. Say you're doing a pediatrics rotation at SickKids Hospital in Toronto, or you're learning about liver failure in pre-clerkship, there are layers of the social determinants of health that are so key to the understanding of these things. I'll give you an example: in a foundational lecture talking about liver failure, one can actually talk about how diseases like hepatitis C and alcoholism tend to be more prevalent in certain populations with specific socio-economic backgrounds.

As I've gone through training, I've learned to approach the ailments of the social determinants as diseases. Diseases of poverty, diseases of income – these actually impact health outcomes. In the palliative care spectrum, you see the cumulative effect of diseases to the social determinants. In 2014, Canadian Press reported on a chart review in British Columbia that showcased that being homeless cut a person's lifespan by 50 per cent. Not 5, 10, or 25 per cent. Extreme homelessness and poverty cut the person's lifespan by 50 per cent. Now I often challenge people: can you name a disease that will cut your life by 50 per cent? Sure, there are young people who have terminal illnesses and genetic disorders, but they tend to be not so frequent. Homelessness is an example of a terminal diagnosis of the social determinants of health; it's a palliative diagnosis. When layered onto chronic diseases and other life-limiting illnesses, it really means our patients are suffering symptomatically and are likely to have higher mortality rates and lower life expectancies.

And so back to your question. As I went through my training, I started to respect the social determinants so much that I now deem them as conditions that I think we should be considering on a medical history, for example, listing high blood pressure, high cholesterol, food insecurity, vulnerably housed, and addictions. I can see that becoming the norm one day.

JK: That's a really strong image, to imagine the cumulative life impact of the social determinants.

ND: In the theory of upstream thinking, the totality – the cumulative effect of the determinants – on individual patients or a population is an opportunity to tell a story about what happens when there is a widening disparity gap in Canada. This is what happens when we don't have Housing First. This is what happens when we don't follow a harm-reduction protocol. And by telling these stories, by supporting the population, we can have upstream interventions that can prevent future populations from going through these. A lot of people ask me why I do what I do. And sometimes the answer surprises them. The answer is that with upstream work, we will have an effect, so that in the future people will not have to deal with these diseases of social determinants the way they currently do.

JK: How do you specifically address upstream efforts through your work?

ND: Clearly, when working on the palliative spectrum of disease, we see the cumulative effect of social determinants, but it doesn't mean that upstream discussions don't happen. If it's hard to live a life when dealing with social ailments, can you imagine what it's like to die with those ailments? Cancer Care Ontario says that 25 per cent of the financial burden from cancer falls on patients and their families, including medications, home care, and travel. It is data like that that shows us that truly, a social-determinants approach is important, even at the end of the disease trajectory. So what we need to do is approach things from that perspective when caring for patients before we do an intake.

When patients pass away, we have a duty in our program to tell their story. Now in some cases, we tell the story through the media when they come to us and give us an opportunity. We've done documentaries, we've done press pieces, we've done student pieces, we do photography, we do art, we showcase people's letters and poems, we do research, we do a qualitative study. So in this program, every death, while it is a tragic event in itself and we mourn the loss of the patient, what we tend to rally around is that we have a story to tell compassionate and passionate Canadians who really are concerned and care about their plight.

JK: What can we do as a professional community to make physicians more aware of the social determinants? What can we do to make it feel easier to do something about them?

ND: I think that's the crux of the matter: systematic approaches to uptake of information and providing physicians and other care providers with the tools to intervene. One of the tools that one could use is data – big data. In the era of electronic medical records, electronic hospital records, we have databases that can be pinned down to postal code, neighbourhood. One approach really revolves around how we dissect and investigate data sets and big data to tell stories. I think also we need to equip clinicians with the knowledge, understanding, and perspective to really deal with some of the social determinants as real diseases. To do that we need to show them that they can be treated, because physicians are healers. Physicians need to see themselves as individuals who can intervene not only by themselves, but also with their care team. So equipping them with the knowledge that this is a real thing and that it impacts health, and then giving them the tools to treat these social determinant issues is really important. The other thing as a profession is that, given that we are in the trenches, given that we are on the front lines of communities that face social inequities, we need to advocate – to advocate for research, to advocate for education, and to advocate for policy changes at local, provincial, national, and perhaps even international levels to really enact and implement social change around these issues.

■■ **JK:** Our new federal health minister is the first physician in nearly a century to hold this position. She often quotes Rudolf Virchow, the nineteenth-century physician who famously said, "Politics is medicine on a larger scale." Given the link between medicine and politics, what are the political changes in Canada that would lead to greater health? What advice would you give to Minister Philpott?

■■ **ND:** First of all, I think we have a unique opportunity to play out policy changes that could impact millions of Canadians at a population level. The first thing that I would talk about with Dr Philpott is pharmacare, a national pharmacare strategy. I think there is enough evidence now to showcase that at least one in ten Canadians can't afford prescription drugs. So in order to prevent acute care hospitalizations and to prevent the sequelae and complications of chronic disease, an upstream approach would be a pharmacare strategy that could leverage the provinces' purchasing power. The healthcare economic data can support this, in addition to the upstream data around a national pharmacare strategy.

The second thing that I would encourage Minister Philpott to look at is a national housing strategy. It's really interesting and encouraging to see that the previous federal government funded the Chez Soi/At Home Demonstration Housing First project. This was a national, randomized, controlled trial looking at housing as an intervention with homeless and underhoused individuals with mental illness. And the findings have shown that individuals with Housing First do better from a housing perspective, from a health perspective, and society tends to gain from a cost perspective. What we have learned from this national $110-million study is that we are in place to be able to encourage a national housing strategy that could dramatically address one of the social ailments that is so commonly plaguing Canadians.

JK: What does a political culture that produces good health outcomes look like?

ND: A political culture that produces good health outcomes incorporates the voices of the people. It incorporates the voices of our patients, their experiences, their highs, and their lows. It incorporates the voices of survivors, and the lessons learned from the experiences of the deceased. It incorporates the healthcare providers as they do work on the front lines. A political culture that supports good health outcomes incorporates the perspective of innovative visionaries, people who are researching new models of care, pilots around pharmacare or Housing First. It incorporates the voices of health economists who have an understanding of the healthcare system and understand cost-effectiveness within a healthcare system. A political culture that truly supports good health outcomes of patients must incorporate the voices of all those groups. That's the heart, that's the beginning. If that foundation is not put in place then we will be missing the boat.

■■ **JK:** Ontario, Quebec, and Newfoundland and Labrador are provinces with physicians as health ministers. Criticism comes quickly from within the medical profession for these figures, as, like in every public-policy field, there is compromise. One question that I always have is about how the medical profession considers political life. There is a lot of struggle between a physician in administrative power and the profession. Dr Philpott is recognized as being in a position of opportunity. I'm wondering if you think there's anything doctors should be doing to encourage her and others who take on political roles?

■■ **ND:** Every profession has people in it that will decide to pursue politics during their careers. The truth is, to be a physician is to be a political agent of health. You know, Virchow was on to something. Whether it's the front lines of clinical care, or subcommittees in your local clinic or hospital, or larger levels, every physician in Canada has the opportunity to advocate for political change that can better the health outcomes of all Canadians. I don't necessarily think that physicians, organizations, or those that are training should empower us to be politicians, but I think that what has already happened through movements like Upstream is an awareness that we as physicians have an opportunity to enact social change through political advocacy, and that can happen through many routes. Some physicians choose to pursue politics officially, others choose to write letters, or engage in advocacy-based research or education, others in advocacy groups, others post articles or blogs. To engage in social change as profession, we need to be involved with all of those media along with politics. That's how we have been able to raise awareness that tomorrow's physician is way more politically aware of the impact that they can have on the social determinants than ever before.

JK: As someone physicians can look up to and, who is a leader in addressing the social determinants of health, whom do you look to? Who has inspired your work? Whom do you admire?

ND: Where to begin? In 2016, there is no shortage of mentors across this country. I think that as part of my trajectory throughout my career and now as a practising physician, I have been blessed to have innovative thinkers, advocates, and outspoken physicians showcase for me what it means to really characterize humanity with compassion and social change through their work, both clinically and administratively. So I'll pick a few examples: Dr Philpott is such a well-spoken, profound, evidence-based individual utilizing the political sphere to enact social change for Canadians from all walks of life. I really admire that. Meb Rashid and Phil Berger are outspoken physicians who at a time of crisis – when a federal policy was passed concerning the support of refugees – stood up and made it really cool for doctors, medical students, and residents to advocate. I can think of innovative thinkers around model-delivery and research: Gary Bloch from Toronto has served as an incredible mentor of mine in the work that we do. Ryan Meili and the Upstream movement have showcased for me how a cultural movement can engage Canadians in awareness around such important and complicated issues. There are numerous examples across Canada: Jeff Turnbull, Leslie Shanks. I've been so influenced by so many people out there from all walks of life, whether that's been clinically in the trenches, advocacy for marginalized patient populations, starting a cultural movement, or focusing on how a hospital can address the social determinants of health.

◼◼ Chapter 6 ◼◼

A System That Puts Health as Its Ultimate Goal: Stories and Ideas for Change

Monika Dutt (Canadian Doctors for Medicare) – Koray Demir

As I began my medical training two years ago, I was quickly drawn to ideas in global health and upstream action for a healthier Canada. The thought of designing and implementing policy that can improve the lives of people nationwide seemed like the most powerful way to apply what I had begun to learn in medical school. Just as soon as I felt committed to the upstream approach of being a physician, though, a number of doubts began to cross my mind. How would I be able to maintain my clinical skills if I focused on policy work? The idea of upstream action is inspiring, but does it actually work in real life? How much was I romanticizing the idea?

As I considered these questions, I was lucky to have been introduced to Dr Monika Dutt, a role model for many colleagues and myself. Dr Dutt is a family and public health physician based in Cape Breton, Nova Scotia, where she also serves as medical officer of health. She is currently the chair of Canadian Doctors for Medicare, where she leads the organization's efforts to advocate for an accessible and equitable healthcare system. She has worked across Canada, including as deputy medical health officer for northern Saskatchewan and alongside members of Parliament in Ottawa as a researcher in health policy. Most recently, Dr Dutt ran in the 2015 federal election as an NDP candidate, bringing her passionate defence of public healthcare – and pharmacare in particular – to the political stage.

I was excited to discuss concepts such as access to medicines – her area of expertise – as well as a number of social determinants of health, like employment and education. I was fortunate to also have had the opportunity to hear from Dr Dutt about how medical students can orient themselves as health advocates, while striking a balance between being a clinician and policy-maker, answering many of my own questions.

Koray Demir: What do you think are the most important forces that shape the lives and health of your patients?

Monika Dutt: You specifically mention your patients, so I was thinking mainly in terms of people I care for now in Cape Breton. The two things that come to mind are income and community. Income, because this is a place where there is a lot of poverty, lack of employment, and lack of other opportunities, so income is a huge factor that shapes their lives. It's also a close-knit, deep-culture kind of place with a number of Mi'kmaq communities and strong Scottish, French, and Celtic heritages. People really have a strong sense of being a Cape Bretoner, or being part of their First Nations community, so that's another really significant force. People are supported by their communities, or sometimes we lose the support of having family members who might go away, or children who move away, so that's a big shaper of people's health.

KD: In Montreal, I've also had the chance to work in a clinic in an underserved area, and I've seen a lot of people from different backgrounds who may not have had many opportunities when they arrived here. It's very interesting to see how inequality and inequity can really be reflected in people's health. What do you think are the benefits and challenges of working with diverse patient populations like this?

MD: As a physician, the challenge and interesting part of working with diverse populations is being open to learning from your patients. Everywhere I've worked has been with people with different backgrounds than mine, whether it's northern Ontario, northern Saskatchewan, Nunavut, downtown Toronto, or Cape Breton. There are varied backgrounds, and I can't claim to share many experiences with the patients that I've worked with. It's about being open and, as much as I can, not making assumptions. Whatever your background is, even if you think you have something in common with your patients, there is probably a lot that you don't. So you want to be open and learn from them, to take whoever is in front of you, work with what they tell you and what they say.

■■ **KD:** It's inspiring that you've had the chance to work in such diverse places, like Nunavut and metropolitan Toronto. Across your experiences, is there one particular patient story that sticks out for you as being especially representative of the ideas of social determinants and health inequality?

■■ **MD:** The person who sticks out most in my mind is someone I just saw, someone from clinic last week. She had come in crying, in tears, stressed out from her work. She works in a call centre, which is one of the jobs here that hires quite a few people. It's a low-education job; she never finished high school. She hates her job, she works full time, is stressed out from her supervisor, and is a single mother taking care of her son. She tried another job that she liked, but she was only able to get part-time hours, so she went back to this call centre job that she can't deal with emotionally. But because she doesn't have the education, she can't find anything else that's full time, and she can't take any time off work to access that education. She's doing all this to give her son a better life than she has had, so it is this cycle that is really impossible for her to get out of right now. She wants to stay in her home community, and even if she did move, she might not be able to get a job because of lack of education. She is still living in poverty despite working full-time hours and doesn't have a partner to help support her family. This patient has a number of different factors that make it really difficult to figure out how to get out of this situation.

▮▮ **KD:** I'm sure you hear those kinds of stories often in your practice. When I came into medical school, I wasn't completely aware of the idea of health equity, but once I began working in the hospital, I saw how different socio-economic backgrounds and opportunities, like education, or even just the environment you were born into, could influence health. What do you think is the best approach to using these stories for political advocacy on behalf of our patients? How do you think we can be inspired by what we see in clinic and use it to make a difference?

▮▮ **MD:** One of the challenges of thinking of things in terms of advocacy is figuring out where to focus. For example, income is a clear determinant of health that is linked to many other factors, and advocacy around income is something that I have been involved in. Lately, I have been getting involved a lot in political discussions, and so much talk is about jobs and the economy. I've been trying to reframe that because we know that two of the greatest determinants in whether you can participate in the economy are child care and transportation. We need to address those determinants rather than just seeing jobs and the economy as the ultimate outcome, and we need to have these supports in order to have full participation in the economy.

It's all about focusing on an issue that you want to get involved in. There is a risk with public health sometimes, feeling as though you can get involved in a million different issues. My advocacy has tended to be in climate change and housing, and even those are massive issues, but you can pick something to focus on and move some policies forward in those areas.

■■ **KD:** It seems like a lot of people who are starting medical school expect to do a lot of brute physiology and anatomy, so when we get hit with these social topics and we talk about income inequality and the environment, it can seem unintuitive at first. People might think that this isn't "real medicine." Why do you think the social determinants are real medicine, and why are they so important?

■■ **MD:** We know that they have the greatest impact on our health. The Canadian Medical Association's quote is that approximately 25 per cent of our health is determined by the healthcare system, and 50 per cent is from social factors. There are a number of different factors here: how we treat our medical students and how we design our curricula. Even from an evidence-based perspective, if you look at the huge amount of research out there right now, we know that issues outside of the healthcare system have the greatest impact on people's health. If we really want to contribute to the health of our patients, we at least have to incorporate some aspect of the social and economic issues in their lives. The things we can do as a doctor just focusing on the traditional medical aspect are relatively few. That is a bit depressing, but instead we can see it as something wonderful, and that we can be much more effective if we see medicine in a much broader way.

■■ **KD:** As I progress in my training, seeing patients who were going through problems related to health equity inspired me to become more involved in public and global health. Is that part of your story as well? Did you come into medicine knowing that you wanted to run for Parliament and work for political change, or was there a moment that helped put you on that road?

MD: As an undergrad, I did a liberal arts degree at McMaster, which was probably one of the most influential times of my life. I began with a focus on social justice issues, and completed a minor in women's studies, with relatively little science. I did my thesis with a woman named Dr Joanna Santa Barbara, who is a psychiatrist, now in Australia, who was the president of Physicians for Global Survival at the time. It was a really active community in Hamilton at the time, so all of this together motivated me to go into medicine.

Near the end of my training, I knew that I wanted to do a Master of Public Health, and found out quite late about community medicine, the residency program, now public health and preventive medicine. I realized there was an area of medicine where we could combine all of these different interests: the core biomedical sciences as well as all the social factors. It was kind of a progression from undergrad, which hinged on meeting really inspirational people along the way. I ended up going into public health and family medicine, and I am able to combine them in my daily work, which is fantastic. I can do patient care and I can spend the rest of my days looking at community issues and policy issues.

KD: What do you think is healthy public policy, especially in Canada? What does a political culture that produces good outcomes look like to you?

MD: It's a system that puts health as its ultimate goal. You can have a good economic picture and still have income inequality increasing, with greater numbers of people living in poverty. Statistics Canada measures things around community connectedness, but do we ever say as a provincial government that that is what we want to see improve? Or alternatively, we could use the outcome of education or access to child care. If we set specific goals, we might expect positive effects on health and employment. An ideal system considers health in all policies, and importantly uses health to measure the effectiveness of what we're doing. This is happening in places in Canada and around the world, it's not an idea that's out of nowhere. We can use this model and make it better, then apply it on a broader scale.

KD: How can Canada improve in taking this health-focused approach in policy discussions?

MD: At the local level, you have community design: roads, parks, and recreation areas. At the provincial level, there's the design of social services, and how to do that in a way to encourage health and education. At the federal level, we have design of our immigration and housing policies. We tend to see them in silos, but if we used health as a connector between them then we would be designing better policy than we are now.

KD: What steps has Canadian Doctors for Medicare taken to advocate for healthier public policy?

MD: Canadian Doctors for Medicare is an organization that I never thought I would become chair of, and now have become really dedicated to. It's an organization that's focused on the healthcare system, and it's a voice for physicians across the country to be able to work to improve our medicare system in the framework of a single-payer universal system. We are focused on healthcare specifically rather than branching into other determinants of health, but within that field, there is a lot that we can be doing to make our system more equitable.

Pharmacare is one issue that has been a major focus of recent political dialogue. Of course the lack of a pharmacare system affects people who are lower income and in jobs without benefits, but really it impacts all of us. If we had a national pharmacare program, it would help people who are unable to afford their medications. This affects one in five families, more than three million people across the country. We have different campaigns that we have done over time, but this has been one that we really focused on in the last few years.

KD: When people think of Canada, there's the idea that we have a very well-functioning and equitable healthcare system. But it seems as though our system still has some issues to work out, especially with access to medicines. What do you think are some major barriers to equitable access to medicines right now?

MD: A major barrier is lack of action from the former federal government. We have had a lot of provinces speak out in support of pharmacare, including the ministers of health in Ontario and Newfoundland, and different premiers across the country. At the Council of the Federation in June 2015 in St John's, Newfoundland, premiers from across the country signed a pledge for national drug coverage. There is also provincial support, and the provinces have been attempting to bulk-buy medications, but it's not nearly what we could have if there was a comprehensive pharmacare program. Until recently, there has been no federal role at all in discussing the issue, and you know the former government stepped away from healthcare in general. We need commitment at a national level, and we definitely don't have nearly enough yet.

Some people argue that it would be too expensive, but there has been a lot of research, especially in recent months, that shows that it makes economic sense to have national pharmacare. From a health perspective, it definitely makes sense because we end up with a lot of people who are sick and in hospitals who don't need to be, because they don't take their medications. It's really about having that federal voice, having a commitment to healthcare.

KD: Do you have any advice from your experiences for the future social justice-minded physicians of Canada?

MD: I learn from the communities I am in, and I try to find ways that I can contribute as well. When you are new in a place, it's really important to get to know your community, get to know the issues, and then find an area that you can focus on.

Also, look for mentors. There are lots of physicians doing fantastic work, and there is a whole range of inspiring physicians you can connect with and learn from. So much of what has guided me are people that I have admired and found as mentors. They can give you inspiration, especially at times when you get really disillusioned and disheartened by medicine.

▮▮ Chapter 7 ▮▮

A Profound Sense of Responsibility: Thinking Large and Small in the Inner City

Ritika Goel (Advocate for Refugees and the Uninsured) – Zachery Hynes

Dr Ritika Goel is a family physician working with marginalized populations in inner-city Toronto, and a passionate advocate of health equity in Canada through her writing and public speaking. She serves as board member and volunteer physician at the Scarborough Community Volunteer Clinic for the Uninsured, serves on the Ontario College of Family Physicians' Poverty and Health Committee, is a founding member of Students for Medicare, and serves on the board of Canadian Doctors for Medicare.

With her clinic closed for the night and the Toronto International Film Festival just beginning to fill the streets below, we met for this interview at her condo in the somewhat tachycardic heart of downtown.

▮▮ **Zachery Hynes:** Can you tell me a little about your work?

▮▮ **Ritika Goel:** I work in three settings: a primary care clinic, a women's drop-in, and a refugee shelter. My clinical focus is primarily around people experiencing homelessness and migrants who are unable to access healthcare due to their immigrations status.

▮▮ **ZH:** Had you always been thinking about these social issues, or was this something that you first were exposed to in medical school?

▮▮ **RG:** I was first exposed to the idea of doing this kind of work in medical school, but everybody is shaped by their own personal experiences. My understanding of the world and my decision to work in certain spaces is probably shaped by the fact that I am a South Asian woman who came here as an immigrant when I was thirteen. It is shaped by the fact that I grew up in India and East Africa and had an understanding of what inequality looks like in the setting of a low-income country. It is also greatly shaped by the fact that I come from a very loving family and I have always had the sense that everybody should be able to have a good life, and there is no reason that we as a society shouldn't do everything we can to ensure that.

ZH: Thinking about the homeless shelters that serve your patient population, what sort of unique challenges do you see in these patients?

RG: With homeless men, you particularly see the impact of incarceration. You see the impact of a history of multiple physical assaults, and engagement in violence, and being in an environment where it is very important to maintain that you are strong, physically and emotionally. We see a lot of men who have experienced tremendous amounts of childhood trauma by way of emotional, physical, and sexual abuse. But the way that it manifests in the men is quite different from how it manifests in the women. In the men it tends to manifest in closing down and feeling that they can't engage with the world, and having difficulty speaking about the trauma, and turning more aggressive in response to that. Whereas with the women you might see a bit more engagement in sex work, or in a different sort of manifestation in terms of anxiety and depression as opposed to aggression.

The challenges come from trauma, they come from intergenerational poverty, and they come from people being born into a difficult situation and their life continuing in that trajectory. The barriers are not being able to access adequate social assistance, a high-enough minimum-wage-paying job, food security, or safe and healthy housing that is affordable. That's where you see the social determinants of health really play out in these populations.

ZH: Thinking about the social determinants of health, what forces do you see most affecting the health of your patient population?

RG: I would say income and housing are probably the biggest social determinants I see in the general population of homeless men and women. We know that income is the number one determinant of health, and I have certainly seen the impact of even the difference between people being on social assistance, where they are only receiving around $600 a month through Ontario Works, which is welfare, and then we are able to get them onto the Ontario Disability Support Program, and then they are accessing about $1,000 a month.

I think of a young man in his late twenties, of Indonesian background, who has been my patient for a few years now and has bipolar disorder. He always presented to me in a very chaotic manner. I saw him several times when he was manic, either just as he was hospitalized or just after he was hospitalized, and I remember the tremendous difference I saw in him when he got housed. It was incredible; it was like I was seeing a different person. He even said to me, and I was impressed at his insight, "You know, when you saw me before, that was who I had to be, because I was on the street. I was in the shelter. I was living that life. I was using. I was gambling. I was just in that space." Somehow, I think being housed provided him the stability to see himself in a different light and to be able to think of a different life for himself. Even as we talk about bipolar disorder as a disease, we rarely talk about it as something that can be influenced that dramatically by housing.

It makes me wonder how many people we are inappropriately treating. Obviously, pharmaceutical treatment has its place, but how many people would perhaps be doing so much better in their mental and physical health if they just had a place to stay at night?

ZH: It makes me think of triple-therapy, how we wouldn't prescribe one-third of a drug regimen we know to be effective. But in a sense, that's what we're doing by treating an illness like that with pharmaceutical therapy alone.

RG: It's a similar story with patients who are refugee claimants. In Canada, when you arrive and make a refugee claim, you get put into the refugee shelter system, but people are not able to get a work permit for several months. So I see people having just arrived in this new country; they're in a shelter, they're on welfare, they have this refugee claim, and they don't know what is going to happen. When their claim has been accepted, and they've gotten housed, they have a work permit, and now they're starting to work, and they're starting to get their permanent residency with a plan to bring their family over – it's an incredible transformation in the levels of anxiety and insomnia, depression, suicidal thoughts, and even the manifestations of post-traumatic stress disorder (PTSD) like nightmares and flashbacks. You see this dramatic change in people once they know that they are in a safe place that they can now call home permanently, and that they are able to begin their new life. Conversely, you'll see the people whose immigration situation gets dragged out over years and years, and they can't ever feel completely settled and calm because they don't really know what's going to happen. Sometimes the best treatment is getting your immigration status.

ZH: You mentioned the profound impact that you see on your patients' mental health as they find housing or obtain their immigration status. Do you see it also having an impact on their physical health?

RG: Absolutely. A great example of that would be insulin care for diabetes. I had a lovely sixty-four-year-old gentleman who lived in the shelter for about ten years and had a complex medical history: on insulin, on Warfarin [a blood thinner], history of coronary artery disease and stroke, and so on. He was getting his medications daily, dispensed by the nurses at the shelter, because he was in a very high-service shelter relative to most places. Unfortunately, due to some issue that occurred at the shelter, he ended up getting discharged, and so now he was on the street. This is a man who for ten years had not injected his own insulin, and now is carrying around his glucometer, his needles, and all his medications, and going from shelter to shelter, and just not taking his medications because he has nowhere to put them. If you think about how most shelters operate, you have to leave during the day, and you come back at a certain time for check-in to make sure that you have your bed, and in many shelters maybe you don't have the same bed every night. Maybe you have to leave your belongings in a locker, or some people carry their belongings around with them. It is incredibly common for people to have their belongings stolen, and for people to be attacked and robbed, particularly if they have any kind of narcotic medications or anything that is addictive in any way. It's difficult to organize your life if you don't have a home base. Managing medications is a potentially fatal example if you just don't have a clean place where you can sit and administer them properly.

ZH: This loss of a sense of place, and a sense that you have a home base, sounds as though it would be very dehumanizing as well.

RG: That speaks to why people are so thankful when you treat them well, because they are perhaps not accustomed to that. I have one patient who refuses to go inside all year long. He sleeps outside. He has slept outside for nearly two years now. He doesn't even come into the shelter because shelters are often not seen as safe places. He is a bit on the older side; he worries about the younger guys taking advantage of him. He is perhaps my only patient who actually chooses to be homeless. In his case, it is because he experienced such a traumatic event related to the last home he was in that he feels unable to get housing again because he has so much fear around what could happen. It has been incredible for me getting to know him and having that human connection with him in a clinic setting, but then also seeing him on the street where he sleeps, and understanding that so many of us walk by so many people who sleep on the street. Actually knowing what someone like that is going through, and why they are where they are, and what it is that would actually help somebody in that situation is quite humbling.

ZH: I often have wished I could do something when I see people on the street who appear to be homeless. I have often heard that many of the things that might initially spring to mind may be more harmful than helpful. I suspect a lot of people who would like to do something, they don't want to do harm, but they don't know how to do good either. Do you have any thoughts on that?

RG: What I suggest doing is advocating for systemic policy change. Sometimes those things get disconnected for people, but remembering that the person on the street that you wish you could help could potentially be helped by you reaching out to your elected representative and saying that we need more affordable housing units. It's really important to keep in mind those interactions that you have with people who might be struggling in some way, and remember what you can do with your power, as a part of society, to improve their life.

ZH: I have become increasingly aware of how much good and harm can be done by policy. In my career as a physician, I may have an impact on thousands of lives over thirty or forty years. In just a few minutes, policy can change that many, or even many more, lives. It's often made me reconsider how I should spend my time as a physician: to what degree should it be political, rather than clinical, if I want to have the greatest impact?

RG: It's true: physicians have an incredible amount of privilege. We are in the top 1 per cent of income earners. We are considered highly respected, highly credible members of society, we have this incredible access to people's lives, and we have this ability to see the impact of policy in a very real way that others don't have. If we truly want to make a difference in health, we have to recognize that the way to do that is through systemic policy change.

There's a campaign right now to push for national pharmacare. When I think about why I want to push for national pharmacare, I think of so many patients I know who have struggled because they have been caught in the loopholes between coverage. Physicians need to recognize that we can channel the stories we know and we can make that impact. We will see it in our work. A national pharmacare strategy – I would see the effects of that the next day in clinic.

ZH: You've done a lot of writing and speaking on these issues. Have you been involved in this sort of thing from an early age?

RG: No, I was a fairly uninformed teenager and adolescent. I have been fortunate in medicine to find really incredible peers and really incredible mentors. I had a great fear of public speaking as a child, although I always enjoyed writing. One of the things that tends to happen in this society is that we give platforms to certain people who look a certain way, and maybe are older, or who tend to be men. I am also very aware of the fact that someone who looks like me may not have been given the space that I have been given if I was not a physician. So I feel a certain responsibility from that perspective of making sure that I am representing voices that are absent in important spaces.

ZH: Can you think of a specific example or experience that particularly contributed to your becoming involved in this sort of work?

RG: When I was in medical school, I heard about the Special Diet clinics. A group of doctors in Ontario were setting up clinics to complete something called the Special Diet form for patients living on social assistance. This was in response to a program that the government provided for people who were on social assistance to get access to funds if they had certain medical conditions. The perspective the physicians were coming from was that living in poverty puts you at risk for many medical conditions.

As a medical student, I worked along with some of these physicians. I did the histories and helped complete some of the forms. It was incredibly inspirational to see some of my supervisors taking this really brave and bold action that was impacting the social determinants of health of the person sitting in front of them, while making this big political statement around how income was an important determinant of health, and how we wanted to do something about it.

ZH: What would a political culture that produces good health outcomes look like?

RG: It would be a political culture where we put people before profits, where we think about the health of a population as a goal. The way to get there is through the population putting pressure on people in power, because people in power won't do anything unless you make them.

ZH: How do we get physicians inspired to believe that they can bring about this sort of change?

RG: We're already starting to see that. I've seen a huge shift between now and when I was in medical training. We're talking a lot more about advocacy and recognizing it as one of the CanMEDS roles that we expect trainees to fulfill. The younger generation of trainees and physicians already gets it. I definitely see that energy and that desire among the newer, younger generation of physicians and trainees.

It's really important for us to be having these discussions in classrooms. Medical school is a place where you go through very rigorous training, you have to read a lot, and you're very busy. People who might be interested in policy/advocacy find each other and find spaces to discuss these things. But this needs to be part of training. We need to be talking about not just social determinants of health in an academic manner, but (1) how you impact social determinants of health within a clinical encounter, and then (2) how do we set up our practices, how do we set up our systems in a way that takes into account those things, and then (3) how do you get involved at that broader policy/advocacy level? If students, residents, and early-career physicians see their mentors doing that, then that's what they'll do.

ZH: You mentioned incorporating the social determinants into clinical practice. This idea translates easily and intuitively to primary care. It's much more challenging for people who are in other

90

kinds of residencies, such as my own field, anesthesia. How do I incorporate that? How do other specialists incorporate this?

■■ **RG:** We have a poverty and health session that we run for medical students at the University of Toronto. We do two such sessions: one in third year and one in fourth year. It's a small-group session that is co-facilitated by a physician and a person with lived experience of poverty. We have that individual share his or her life story, and then we go through cases. I had to keep shifting gears in my mind about how to ensure that the students around the table who were going into different specialties were able to see their role. The first thing that everybody can do is just treat patients well. That might seem like a really easy thing to do, but it's certainly not an experience that a lot of marginalized patients have in the healthcare system. For example, if you see an individual come in who seems to be under the influence, or maybe they appear dishevelled, and they're coming in with some sort of a physical health complaint, do not simply assume that their physical health complaint is related to a mental health issue; take them seriously and validate them.

Other great examples: if you are working on an inpatient unit – medicine, surgery, whatever it is – recognize that a lack of housing will impact a person's post-operative care. It will impact the outcome of the pneumonia they've been admitted for. Or learning about the community services in your area, and then finding, as we are lucky to have in Toronto, an infirmary program that takes in homeless individuals for a few days for convalescent care, and recognizing the impact that that can make in people's health outcomes. It's about, wherever you are in the healthcare system, learning how to assess a person's social situation, and recognizing how their social situation is going to impact their health outcome.

Another classic example is medication coverage. Too often I have a patient either discharged from hospital, or who sees a specialist, and then is sent home with a prescription for very expensive medications that are either not covered by the public drug plan, or the patient doesn't have any drug coverage. These expensive medications could have easily been substituted with cheaper medications in the same class. Recognizing that a person's low income affects their drug coverage, and altering your actions in a way that they will actually be able to fill your prescriptions and follow through on your recommendations, is a very tangible way that you can improve people's health outcomes. The most recent numbers say one in five people in Canada don't fill a prescription due to cost. So all those beautiful prescriptions we're writing out, and all that wonderful knowledge we've got about what is first-line and second-line, and thinking about the side effects and allergies – for one in five people, that is useless.

ZH: You write, you speak, you care for patients in a clinic and you volunteer. What sustains you through all of this busyness?

RG: What sustains me is probably just a profound sense of responsibility. I couldn't be comfortable not doing anything, knowing what I have, and what others don't have, and knowing that I have the power to do something to change that. How could I not? The problem that I usually have is stopping; the problem is not with doing things.

◼◻ Chapter 8 ◼◻

Every Clinical Story Has a Social Story

Brian Goldman (CBC's *White Coat, Black Art*) – Andrew Bresnahan

Dr Brian Goldman has worked as an emergency physician at Mount Sinai Hospital in Toronto for more than twenty years. He is known across Canada as CBC Radio One's house doctor, and is the host of their award-winning show White Coat, Black Art. *The show guides listeners through the culture of medicine, exploring topics as diverse as pharmacare, home births, physician-assisted dying, cue jumping, user fees, empathy and physician burnout, racism in healthcare, and what makes a good doctor.*

The bestselling author of Night Shift: Life in the ER *and* The Secret Language of Doctors, *he is also a prolific public speaker. Over one million people have viewed his TED talk, "Doctors make mistakes – Can we talk about that?" He is at once a front-line doctor and a storyteller, exploring the source of patient and physician experiences in a changing health system.*

When Dr Goldman and I met up, I'd just flown south from Nunatsiavut, the Inuit homeland on Labrador's north coast, where I was born and now work as a resident physician. While Dr Goldman's emergency room in Toronto is in many ways a world away from the communities where I learn and work as a rural generalist, I've realized we tackle many of the same challenges, both as physicians and as storytellers. In Toronto and Nunatsiavut alike, every clinical story has a social story.

◼◻ **Andrew Bresnahan:** How do your experiences as a physician and journalist inform your thinking on the social determinants of health, the conditions of everyday life that shape people's health?

▌▌ Brian Goldman: First of all, I work in an emergency department, so let's start with patients. I see people who suffer the consequences of failing to address the social determinants of health. And when I say failing, I don't mean they failed; I mean that there is a failure somewhere – maybe it's a combination of failures. For instance, I work in a hospital in downtown Toronto where we see lots of homeless people. We see lots of people with substance abuse. We see lots of people at the margins of society. Clearly, they are not benefitting from having their social determinants of health satisfied – having a roof over their head or an education. Where they live clearly determines their fate to a large extent. I see patients who are overweight, who smoke cigarettes, who drink alcohol, three of the major risk factors for most of the chronic diseases we see that soak up seventy-five cents out of every dollar of healthcare expenditures. Very often in the emergency department what I'm doing is putting out fires, patching the end results of not addressing the social determinants of health.

As a journalist, I see it more on a society-wide scale. For instance, recently on my show *White Coat, Black Art*, we did an entire episode devoted to "vaping," or e-cigarettes, inhaling vapour of nicotine instead of nicotine plus tobacco products. What we got to see was an industry developing to help people transition away from tobacco to e-cigarettes. That's an example of trying to mitigate harm by transitioning people from one vehicle to another. What we see there is not addressing one of the key determinants of health, but trying to mitigate the damage. In my medical journalism, I'm constantly citing statistics on rates of cancer, rates of stroke, so I see that and I don't see it going away. Occasionally, we do have people on the program who look at social determinants of health, but the perception in the public is that that's not very interesting. People are much more interested in the latest treatment for cancer than they are in addressing the social determinants of health. It's boring to them, because it's stuff that we take for granted.

We did more than one show on medical geography, on hotspots, on the difference in the health profile of different neighbourhoods. As Andrew Pike says, you can learn quite a lot about someone's health by learning their postal code.

■■ **AB:** In medicine, we have a chance to witness how these patterns are experienced on a human scale. Too often, we see the downstream consequences of upstream failures. What do you think makes for successful storytelling or communication on these themes? How can we share these stories in a way that inspires understanding and action?

■■ **BG:** There's certainly a lot of interest these days in narrative medicine, helping to support patients as they figure out and tell their own stories. There's no question that we're hard-wired to be a storytelling people. We use metaphorical language to talk about patient experience. Certainly for people who work in healthcare, seeing patients as not simply a disease but as a person helps us see what their challenges are and how they've gotten to where they are, both in terms of their health and in terms of their attempt to change their life script so that their health takes a turn for the better. So one thing you can try to do is get inside the heads of the people you're talking about. Instead of looking at them as an object of disease, stand beside them and try to find out from them the view from where they are. They may be in a deep pit looking up at the top, seeing how difficult the journey is. Seeing the hospital from the patient's point of view is really interesting. The best way to tell a story is to establish whose story it is you're telling. Sometimes it will be the health professional's story, trying to help people in a system that won't let them. Sometimes the story is about the patient, and the health professional is a helper or hinderer. Ultimately, if you want people to read your stories or relate to them, they have to see themselves in the story.

■■ AB: That takes concepts that might otherwise be abstract, especially things like epidemiological statistics, and humanizes them, doesn't it?

■■ BG: Journalistically, we sprinkle statistics in here and there. There's a moment when you tell the personal story, and then you pull back to see the landscape. How many people like "George" are there? One of the things I've seen health professionals do is just recite tons of statistics, and they don't even know why, or they put them in because there's a little section in every paper called "epidemiology." So they do a recitation of studies, without editorializing. But in the world of journalism, which is really storytelling, it's a statistic with a purpose.

Yesterday, I did my weekly column on CBC Radio on something that's kind of disturbing at first blush, fraught with ethical issues. It was a survey of oncologists in the US published last week in the *Journal of Clinical Oncology* that found that half of respondents said they had been taught to recognize potential donors in their patients. A third of them were actually asked by their hospitals to ask patients to be donors. Of those who'd been asked, half said yes, half said no. So I began my introduction to the column with the statistic that 200,000 people will be diagnosed with cancer this year, and at least half of them will be alive in five years. That's a lot of grateful patients. So I used the statistic as an entry point to the story.

So very quickly it becomes a question of how you would feel if, at the end of successful treatment, you're in remission and your doctor asks you to become a donor. Does this make you happy? Would you be grateful? Could you say no? So I put myself into the position not of being the doctor asking someone to donate, but rather of the patient or family member who might be quite startled or put off by that.

AB: How does reframing the story this way change it for you?

BG: The show started as pulling back the curtain and revealing what we as doctors think. The heartbeat of the show is how that thinking impacts patients. I'm talking with listeners who are not primarily a medical audience, so I act as a guide, like a curator of what goes on in hospitals. Just as on a safari, a guide might say, "These are the wildebeests, and this is what they do," I'm saying, "These are the medical oncologists, and this is what they do." I'm taking them on a trip through the hospital. The doctors don't like this idea because it could compromise our relationship with the patients, because suddenly there's a shift in the purpose of the doctor-patient relationship. Maybe the purpose now is a donation. Will there be disappointment if the patient says no? Will the patient feel comfortable saying no?

AB: I was just listening to your town hall on pharmacare with Danielle Martin and others. You had a panel of remarkable folks up on stage, bringing a lot of expertise to bear. But I noticed that you always came back to the experiences of the patients, and it kept the conversation accountable.

BG: You always have to come back to the patient. There are questions you can ask that have a direct bearing on a patient, like "Why do we have the most expensive generic drugs on earth?" And that's a bit abstract, but in an essay you can afford to ask the "why" questions. Your average listener will understand that they are paying way more for brand names. The way the world works, you go from brand names to generics and you expect to get a big windfall, and in Sweden they do. In Canada we don't. And that's important, because that affects your pocketbook. That also affects what your government pays for drugs, which means it's going to affect your taxes.

AB: It's fascinating that you bring up Sweden because, of course, it's a country that's done a lot to address social determinants of health. Sweden's social democracy includes investments in public transportation, employment security, child care, maternity and paternity leave. It's kind of wonderful that we live in a world where this natural experiment is taking place. We're not alone. We can look at how other people have tried to tackle these problems. Can you think of any examples where you've seen something another country has done in terms of upstream action and thought, "This is something we could do"?

BG: Sweden's a great example. I was just there and it's fresh in my mind. I spoke with a midwife who is part of a health/human resources approach that's completely flipped the paradigm that we have here in Canada. There are parts of Canada where 80 per cent of all births are attended by obstetricians. In Sweden, 70 per cent are attended by midwives. How does it work? They are part of the system; they work in conjunction with an obstetrician. Family doctors aren't involved at all; it's just midwives and obstetricians. They have midwifery as an established profession, with a midwifery college, probably one of the first in the world, going back to something like the 1700s. That's an interesting national experiment.

Another interesting fact: in Canada, I've met midwives in Montfort

Hospital in Ottawa, a francophone hospital, and there the midwives are starting to attend higher-risk births, they're attending breech births. That used to be considered a complete no-no in Canada, and they're doing it and they're doing it successfully. So I asked a midwife I was talking to in Sweden, "Are you doing it here?" expecting the answer would be yes, and she said no, a study a few years ago showed higher complication rates, so they backed off completely. Midwives know their scope of practice, and they're risk-averse. When we think of pushing the frontiers of medicine, you don't think of retreating, you think of pushing them forward. What would it take for them to switch back? She lamented that now midwives don't know how to do it, because it's had a negative reinforcing effect – the more you worry about it, the more you're skittish, you're sensitized looking for risk and complication, and you back off some more and some more, and before you know it you're not doing it at all. And here, halfway around the world, we have midwives here in Ottawa who think "Why not?" and are doing it, in a setting where midwifery is virtually non–existent.

Sweden has a broad social safety net and higher taxes. The marginal tax rate's highest margin was just raised to 50 per cent, so you have people saying, "What do I want to make another $1,000 for if the government is going to take $500?" But, they flirted with lower taxes when they had a right-of-centre government eight or ten years ago, that ran and won on a platform of lower taxes, and when they experienced the reduction in services and programs, they said, "Nah, I don't need a few extra dollars in my pocket, the tax cut wasn't worth it."

■■ **AB:** When we see that we're getting something from taxation, we're more likely to support it than when we're dealing with systems and services that have been chronically eroded.

▮▮ BG: We're on a pendulum. The zero point of the pendulum in Sweden is very different than Canada. We may be destined to have lower tax rates than Sweden and lower quality of services, and more of everybody for themselves. There's talk that we're entering a conservative century, a striver's century, where as long as I can take care of my own, I want more tax dollars back in my pocket. I want fewer services; let the others take care of themselves. In Sweden, they don't do that. In Sweden, their philosophy is that together we can do more than separately.

Going back to the latter days of the Martin government, we've had a good solid ten years of "Wouldn't it be nice to have more money in your pocket? We're the most overtaxed nation on earth," which is ridiculous – we're not. A few targeted boutique tax credits here or there, is that going to make you feel better? Maybe it will. A little extra money in your pocket, a thousand dollars, but a thousand dollars disappears pretty quickly. We've gone through a ten- or twelve-year period of dreaming small. We're starting to dream a little bigger now. What could this country do that's greater?

▮▮ AB: All of this reminds me of Rudolf Virchow, the great nineteenth-century physician who's considered the founder of both cellular pathology and social medicine. He zoomed in on the minutiae of biology, while famously observing that "medicine is a social science, and politics is but medicine on a larger scale." As a physician and storyteller, what do you think are the most important political changes we can make to improve the health of Canadians?

▮▮ BG: Let's go back to the social determinants: raising the education level. Raising the health-literacy level. Rewarding people for taking care of their health – I'd rather give a tax cut to someone who goes from being unfit to being fit, and not just reward someone who's already doing it. Evening out discrepancies in wealth. Having good social networks of friends. Making it easier for people to care for each other when things are tough by paying a salary to those unpaid caregivers. Those are the kinds of things I think we should do.

You're probably familiar with the adverse childhood experiences study in the US from the Centers for Disease Control that found the common factor with addictions to food, alcohol, and tobacco is early childhood trauma. I don't know how you address that, but it's an important piece of information. Trying to address it at age sixty is probably too late.

AB: When we're talking social determinants of health, we're also in a way talking about the capacity to strive, right? It's hard to live up to your full potential if you're waking up hungry, or if your parents are coming home stressed from working two jobs. This relates to how we frame these conversations about health and about politics and about social justice.

BG: And I'm not tossing middle-aged and older adults into the ashcan – there are things that can be done for them. I've been taking a good hard look at harm reduction. If vaping turns out to be better than tobacco, then get them off tobacco and onto vaping. If you save lives by doing that, then do it. It's a band-aid, but we've got to do something.

The other thing is, if someone missed those classes on health literacy because they were established in 2017 and they're sixty, seventy, eighty years old, I think what we could do is hook them up with health coaches. I'm really intrigued by the possibility that a health coach – as an entry-level job, not a profession – could be a peer counsellor. The model is from addictions counselling. Who are the best people to teach you? Not the doctor or the nurse practitioner who's wagging their finger, saying you need to quit, but rather somebody who's been through that journey, who knows what it's like, who understands that it's a lifelong affliction. A health coach is a peer, someone who knows a little bit more than you, a little like that smart family member you wish you could bring with you to the clinic who knows all the right questions to ask, who after you leave the doctor's office with the prescription can say, "Let's make sure you fill it, let's make sure you know how to take it," and who calls you the next day and says; "So how's that going? Are you getting any side effects?" There's a company in the US called Iora Health. What they do is double the amount they spend on primary care and take a corresponding amount away from acute specialist care, and use that money to pay for health coaches, primarily – a few more doctors, but it's not doctor-centric, because this broken model of primary care has doctors spending ten minutes with a patient. What are you going to accomplish with ten minutes?

■■ AB: That's interesting to me, because it seems that the health coach would need to be supported by a broader team too, that's engaging these other problems. Most of these determinants can't be changed by willpower alone, which challenges the idea that if only we had better behaviour we'd have better health outcomes. The thing that rescues the idea of a health coach to me is the notion that maybe they'd have an intimate understanding of the constraints that someone is working with.

■■ BG: They would know, for instance, that grandma didn't fill her prescription because maybe she doesn't know how to arrange for delivery and can't leave the house because she's looking after her single-mother daughter's two kids who are in preschool. What doctor is going to know that or have the time to unpack that? Or maybe there's a language barrier, and she can't find a pharmacy with a pharmacist who speaks her language. Those are the connect-the-dots details that are make or break.

AB: And they're the details we can sometimes miss even when we carry tremendous expertise in medicine. You're a smart guy, you have expertise and interest, and you're in practice. Do you still encounter patients who effect a big shift in the way you think about things?

BG: Yes, and often they are the difficult ones, the ones who make life difficult for you. I remember being dressed down by the husband of a patient I saw who had died. There was no problem with my care; there was a problem with my caring. I did my job, I referred her to internal medicine, but he wanted me to see that this woman who had been the centre of his family was on her last legs, and he was right. He was right. So I had a meeting with him and his family, and I listened, and I started to cry, because that could have been my mom.

We often shut that off. We're not bad pcople. I'm not a bad person. We'rc all part of each other's larger stories, and maybe at that moment I could have responded better but didn't. I had trouble being patient because I was under stress in the emergency department. One of the things I like to do on the show is connect those dots and give some thought bubbles to show what people are thinking when something goes wrong. For instance, on that occasion it might have been that I made the referral to internal medicine to admit her, which was the right thing to do, but I'd already referred three other patients to the medical resident, who'd given me a progressively harder and harder time with each one and was giving me the third degree. So knowing what I had to do filled me with dread and anxiety that I was going to be dressed down again – there's got to be an easier way to make a living than dealing with a human being who's giving me a hard time or making me feel stupid for making a referral. This is what happens when we don't empathize with each other. I try to do that in my better moments.

I'm not always perfect. I was seeing a patient with chronic pain, a smart patient; she talked about how long she'd had to wait. And so I reorganized my schedule and left more time between my patients.

The triumphs don't teach you anything. They're worth savouring, they keep you warm on cold nights, but the grist for the mill are the failures, the mistakes, the moments when you weren't at your best.

▌▇ AB: Taking care of ourselves and each other is as important at a personal level as it is at a broader social level. What are some things that you do to sustain yourself in your work, to keep your ability to empathize with others intact?

▌▇ BG: One of the things I do is keep variety. The fact that I'm not absolutely full time in medicine and not absolutely full time in journalism allows me to use one to buttress the other. On my worst days as a doctor, I remember that I host a radio show; on my worst days as a radio show host, I remember that I'm an emergency physician.

I talk, I share, I reveal what I'm feeling, and I encourage others to do that. I reflect. I write. That's cathartic for me. I also have my guilty pleasures: I love watching films and pure escapist TV shows. I like good storytelling, because I see the stories in others and I've written stories myself, and I like it when it's done well, and it gives me pleasure. It's part of what makes our existence on earth bearable, something to look forward to.

▮▮ Chapter 9 ▮▮

A New Vision for Our Planet and Our Health

Courtney Howard (Canadian Association of Physicians for the Environment) – Kelly Lau

Dr Courtney Howard is a proud mom, dancer, and physician hailing from North Vancouver who has spent the last few years hospital-hopping around Canada, working in ERs in British Columbia, Ontario, Quebec, and the Northwest Territories. She is a board member of the Canadian Association of Physicians for the Environment and has worked with Médecins Sans Frontières/Doctors Without Borders in Djibouti. She practises family and emergency medicine in Yellowknife, and has been one of the key drivers of the climate change and health movement, including leading the latest successful campaign for divestment of fossil fuels by the Canadian Medical Association.

The first time I was in touch with Dr Howard was via email; however, soon enough, after I expressed my interest in health environmental issues, she took the time to speak with me via Skype from snowy Yellowknife. Her humour and passion for social justice was evident when discussing our shared interest in social justice and environmental stewardship. My prior work in environmental health advocacy was only bolstered through her work on climate change and health.

▮▮ **Kelly Lau:** How did you first become interested in the social determinants of health?

▮▮ **Courtney Howard:** At first I'm not sure if I knew what the term meant, but after having worked a variety of different locums, including the Far North and some training in Vancouver in the Downtown Eastside, I think it became clear. When I was working in those environments, some patients were set up to have good health outcomes, and others faced much greater health challenges. I've also worked internationally with Doctors Without Borders, which is how I ended up in the North in the first place. It was really my mission with them in Djibouti in 2011 – working on a pediatric malnutrition project – that led me to understand that my international health interest ties into my work in climate change.

I remember being very aware of social determinants when I was going to my first locum in Inuvik. I was in the Edmonton airport and it was right after twelve years of studying medicine, so I was very conscious of the fact that I knew absolutely zero about the rest of the world. I had made an effort to read broadly – I made a file on my computer called "geeky learning about the world." So I was at the Edmonton airport, and one of the airport stalls was selling a book about the oil sands. I didn't know anything about it, but I was going north and, of course, the Mackenzie River runs right through Inuvik downstream from the oil sands so I figured I should know something about it. This was my first introduction to the concept of an environmental crisis, and I found it extremely upsetting.

■■ **KL:** What was the most worrying part of it?

■■ **CH:** I had written some climate/health articles for the David Suzuki Foundation before going to Djibouti, and even then, I found the environmental data worrisome. It filled me with a sense of concern that this topic didn't seem to be addressed by people whom I had regarded as my medical elders. I guess it was the first major health problem that I didn't think a grown-up was taking care of. So, after my work with the David Suzuki Foundation, I went to Africa. It was difficult to tell if there was a climate component when working there because no one could find any climate data for the country. The NGOs who were working on water couldn't figure it out, but the camels and goats weren't doing very well and there was definitely a migration of people from rural areas to urban centres. That being said, one of the major causes of the food crises was the increase in food prices in 2008, and those increases had more international reasons than local reasons.

Around the same time, there was a malnutrition crisis in the Sahel that was known to have a climate component. But it was really at the bedside after one of the children had died, after the mother thanked me for the care, when it hit me. It is such a heartbreaking feeling after you have just lost a patient – here is this displaced woman who didn't even have the papers to become a refugee from Somalia who just thanked me for my care. I was just filled with such rage at the death of this little person. I promised that once I'd come back to Canada, I'd do everything in my power to prevent similar deaths.

For me, it was just one of those searing moments. I knew that in order to remain whole as a human, I was going to have to make sure that I fulfilled that promise. And when I came back to Canada, right before the malnutrition crisis in Somalia, I really wanted to go back. But by then I was pregnant and couldn't, even though I was extremely motivated to do so. As I tried to reintegrate into life in Canada, in my very privileged world where many of my contemporaries felt that if it isn't organic, it isn't acceptable for their children. (I respect that decision – I buy a lot of organic food myself.) It was just a very huge transition for me. I was very conscious of the inequality in the world, but unable to return to work directly because of family commitments. I was really seeking a way to honour the concerns of the patients I had taken care of overseas while also honouring the experiences of Canadians and the needs of my own family.

It's easy to get angry with people for things that they know nothing about, and that's not fair. It's not fair to get mad at people in Canada for not knowing about how bad it is in other places because they haven't necessarily had the opportunity to see that.

Working full-out on climate change and health seemed to me the best way I could contribute to the health of people at home, overseas, and to my own family. Especially given that Canada won the "Fossil of the Year" award seven times [given to the country doing the most damage to climate talks in a given year].

KL: We are probably one of the worst countries both in terms of our privilege and inaction toward climate change.

CH: The upside to inaction is there is a lot of potential for massive change. Given our natural resources, our solar, wind, and well-educated workforce, we have a ton of room to move and with the right incentives could quickly go from climate laggard to climate leader.

KL: What are some of the most important forces shaping the lives of your patients in Yellowknife? Are you able to see the link between climate change and health?

CH: It was not part of a coherent plan that I developed an interest in climate change and health, and that my husband and I moved up to the North. He had done some of his training up here; he is a pediatrician and found there was a great pediatrics job here. I joined the emergency practice, so we had already planned to move to Yellowknife before I even went to Africa, and then it just happened that we were here right when I developed this interest.

Of course, we are already two degrees warmer in Yellowknife than before. We are one of the canaries in the coal mine when it comes to seeing health effects of climate change. We are seeing decreased reliability of ice roads on lakes and rivers, which act as the main way to get around up here in the winter. That has real consequences for our patient population in terms of their ability to access land-based traditional foods as well as to socialize and have the ability to visit people.

The wildfires that we had in summer 2014 were terrible. Here in Yellowknife, the air quality was so bad that we topped out the air quality health index multiple times over the course of the summer, and PM2.5 levels [minute particles that can enter the lungs and even the bloodstream] were astronomical; that lasted for two-and-a-half months, off and on. People were talking about the summer that never was, because if you follow the recommendations for air quality index, really we shouldn't have been outside for a whole part of the summer. And that's after having spent a whole winter inside. So we had a lot of asthmatics in emergency and lots of people showing up with cabin fever. There was a general sense of malaise and frustration in the town for most of the summer, so that kind of spurred our work looking into the health effects of that summer, spearheaded by Dr James Orbinski.

KL: So you mentioned the mother in Djibouti and some other cases that you encountered working in Yellowknife. What are some of the narratives that keep you going? What drives you to continue your advocacy work?

CH: The malnutrition project that I was working on looked like a bunch of big tents with rows of beds and moms on each bed. Many of these mothers were displaced people, with very little in terms of resources and very little ability to turn the wheels of this system. I'm very conscious of my privilege as a woman at a moment in time where my voice can be heard. I feel a real responsibility not to waste that, to represent the interests of those who just haven't had the same training that I have.

Secondly, I think it's the responsibility that *The Lancet* talked about in their 2015 Climate Change and Health Commission. If it was all doom and gloom, I would be off in an earthship tomorrow, but I really am pleased by the incredible potential that we have for us to leave our children in a much more liveable world. What are the chances that we are alive when the science is there, that bad things are going to happen (we are feeling it in our bodies, through storms and fires and droughts), and at the same time we have just developed the technology required, at the right price, to potentially get us out of a large part of the mess? What are the chances?

We are right in the middle of it – what a great movie plot. It's the most incredible plot line pivot point of human history. And bringing the focus to a shared concern for human health has the ability to shift the pivot. Who better to talk about that than physicians? As physicians right now in Canada, we are the best-equipped, most well-placed people to give the best rationale for the most important health issue of our time, in a country that probably has the biggest potential for change of any in the world. How often do you find yourself in that position?

KL: Agreed, it's a unique problem since this is such a huge health issue, yet so little light has been shed on it until now. Why do you think that is the case?

▎▎ CH: There are a couple of reasons. One, doctors are busy, and this tends to fall in between disciplines. So even though this has been in *The Lancet*, the *British Medical Journal*, and the *American Medical Association Journal*, if you are not looking for it, and you just try to review what is necessary for you in your specialty, you easily could have just not seen the articles. We have lacked champions at a national level who would have helped put this issue in the mainstream, where it needs to be.

Number two, there are really under-recognized mental-health issues with this problem, and physicians are not immune. Because I give presentations on climate change, I am very familiar with the look that physicians get when you get to the bottom line. The bottom line is that we are headed to four degrees Celsius by 2100 on our current emissions trajectory, and we are not expected to adapt effectively to that as a civilization. On hearing that, people look really depressed. There are two options when you get to that point: you either veer off and do something else, or you wade through it until you've reached the point where you have both processed it internally and found some solutions you can work on. The second path is very time-consuming, and it is a lot of work.

My daughter was six months old when I read Bill McKibben's "Terrifying New Math" (*Rolling Stone* magazine, 12 July 2012). I basically was depressed for around six months. It's like suddenly my daughter's future outlook was not as bright as what I thought it was. That was really hard. One of the other physicians in town had something similar happen to him; he didn't get on an airplane for three to five years after he realized what the bottom-line effect of air travel was on climate change. I met a couple other physicians from Ontario online, and they have had the same thing happen to them. Doctors know the science, they tend to be action-oriented, they know what needs to be done, and they see it not being done, so they feel hopeless. They're just trying to live their lives and get over it.

■■ **KL:** It's funny, because I think a lot of medical students who are interested in this issue have also experienced this depression. How can we, as you say, "wade through it"?

■■ **CH:** I found that there is no greater way than through action. I think most physicians who get involved feel that way too. As someone who spends a lot of time on this, which is not available to most doctors, I see my job as becoming excellent at both making a plan and communicating a plan in simple terms.

■■ **KL:** So what do you think is the plan?

■■ **CH:** Right now, the issue of climate change is in the environment box, but people only care about the environment box to a certain extent. Everybody cares about the health box. Study after study, survey after survey, shows that Canadians care about their health. So it is our job to communicate clearly that climate change is in the health box and to take ownership about trying to find solutions.

We need to reinforce and support the people who are making the system. I'm working with an economist who does carbon pricing, and he asked me to work with him because he didn't have the scientific knowledge to talk about climate change. He was trying for years to get carbon price legislation in the territories, but was always unsuccessful because he was never formally trained in anything scientific or environmental. When he learned I had an interest in climate change and health, he asked me to present with him. I looked at carbon pricing for a bit and realized that pretty unanimously, academics – even the head of the World Bank – have been asking for carbon pricing.

Once I realized that this was a dependable thing to support, we put together presentations on "a carbon price for what ails us." I would talk about the health effects of climate change, and everyone would look down and seem to feel a bit depressed. Then I would say, "Hey, now do what Doug says." And so Doug Ritchie would talk about carbon taxes. I liked it because there was a clear action item associated with the presentation instead of people just becoming depressed. Doug liked it because he didn't have to wade into climate science and also because people actually came to his presentation. I mean, who wants to come listen to a presentation about a carbon tax?

KL: How do you think health can act as a rallying force to bring all these multidisciplinary groups together?

CH: The Canadian Association of Physicians for the Environment teamed up with the Ontario Nurses' Association and the Lung Association for the phase-out of coal power in Ontario. I know in that instance, the health voice was key there. Dr Joe Vipond in Alberta has been massively important in leading their coal electricity power phase-out, and that is definitely being done through a health lens. Prior to the 2015 election, he got the four parties to agree to a four-year coal phase-out, so it's policy now.

Urban planners and public health doctors have collaborated well to build healthy, low-carbon environments. There is also a doctor who has been super active in Montreal trying to increase their cycling grid. Doctors are going to city hall meetings when there is a bike lane in discussion, to stand up and present evidence about the health benefits of bike lanes. The New Zealand Land Transport Agency actually calculated how much every kilometre walked by its population, and every kilometre cycled, saved their healthcare system. So can you imagine if we did that comprehensively in healthcare dollars? Can you imagine how that would connect municipal budgets to provincial budgets for healthcare and allow us find out more imaginative ways to fund bike lanes and better transport?

KL: There are so many options for how to address climate change on higher levels. How do you think this will affect our future patients?

CH: I think the more we are able to build healthy, low-carbon, walkable environments, with fresh water and local food, the better everyone is going to feel. The data has shown that the more eyes on the road, the more you are going to chat with your neighbours, the fewer feelings of social isolation, the nicer neighbourhoods you will have, and the better health outcomes you will have in terms of cardiovascular and respiratory disease, etc. Low-cost local foods are more likely to taste good and to have a smaller carbon footprint. I think we need to paint a better picture of where we are going and where we want to get to. We have to start becoming like the condo sellers who show glossy photos of people doing things and walking places instead of scaring people with a ragged, torn, scary future. What motivates you more and makes you want to get out in the world to contribute?

I think the job for Canadian doctors is to (a) learn about climate change, (b) come up with an action plan, and (c) do their best to communicate that plan to their patients. It is amazing when you set the wheels in motion how many people join in.

▮▮ Chapter 10 ▮▮

Recharged: The Energy of a Politically Engaged Physician

Simon-Pierre Landry (Regroupement des médecins omnipraticiens pour une médecine engagée) – Claudel Pétrin-Desrosiers

There aren't many doctors who can juggle caring for a two-year-old child, working in a busy emergency room, running a political campaign, and making numerous media appearances, all while running marathons. Dr Simon-Pierre Landry is one of them.

Trained at the University of Sherbrooke, he pursued a rural residency in British Columbia, where he further developed his taste for emergency medicine. Returning to Quebec in 2012 for his third year of residency, he dove fully into the Printemps Érable: Maple Spring, the Quebec student movement of 2012. And that's when it clicked: he finally connected all his ideas and observations on social inequality and injustice that he'd been trying to understand for years. Every day in his emergency room he would see poverty, vulnerability, and social isolation. He felt he had to do more than consult, and that's why he decided to throw himself into politics. He co-founded an organization of family physicians seeking greater public engagement (le Regroupement des omnipraticiens pour une médecine engagée, or ROME) with the objective of proposing sustainable solutions for a more just health system. He was a candidate for the NDP in the 2015 federal election, putting forward a campaign based on the social determinants of health.

Still at the beginning of his career, Dr Landry certainly has a promising future. Animated by his passion for social justice and public

access to healthcare, he projects a contagious enthusiasm for political engagement. I had the chance to meet him just a few hours before the launch of En Amont, the francophone branch of Upstream. I sensed his unshaken dynamism, his optimism for change, and his will to improve the health of the country.

■■ **Claudel Pétrin-Desrosiers:** Could you tell me about your journey in medicine, your path toward the domain of health and politics?

■■ **Simon-Pierre Landry:** I have been interested in economics and politics since high school, but when I started medicine I wasn't really an activist. When I did my third year in emergency medicine at Charles Le Moyne hospital, I lived through the Printemps Érable. I lived right on the street of the "casseroles" [protest marches animated by banging pots and pans]. And that's when it clicked: 2012 gave me the desire to participate in the movement.

One thing led to another, and particularly because I practise in emergency, it became clear to me that my patients are often marginalized and vulnerable in a way that's disproportionate to the rest of the population. Yes, there are fractures, traumas, car accidents, but most of the patients that come to emergency, and that we see frequently, are marginalized and socially isolated.

I see a lot of poverty in the rural areas, which is different from the type of homelessness and street life that we tend to think of when we speak of typical poverty. I also worked in Yellowknife, where the question of Indigenous health is predominant. It became impossible for me to just "do my shifts." I had to do more, to find the why behind the presenting complaint.

I decided to get involved in politics when Bill 20 was announced by the Quebec government in November 2014. This is when I joined ROME, an organization of which I am now the spokesperson. Bill 20 was an attack on social justice, an attack on women, and a step toward privatization of primary care. [Bill 20 is a controversial omnibus bill that set patient quotas for family doctors working in clinics and hospitals in order to avoid a 30 percent fee cut. The bill also ended public funding for IVF, and allowed doctors to charge an extra fee for a publicly-insured service given in privately-owned clinics.] ROME was developed because we needed a progressive voice in the medical profession to be better allied with the public. Our goal is to have a health system that functions better, and this would require the withdrawal of Bill 20.

I then had the opportunity to become a candidate for the NDP in the 2015 federal election. For my campaign, I proposed a political vision of healthcare based on the social determinants of health. I spent many weeks explaining to people that my power to change things in my emergency room is very limited. We need to act upstream from emergency rooms to attain greater social equity in order to obtain a better level of health for everyone.

That's how I met Ryan Meili, and he told me all about Upstream and the ideas behind that project. Inspired by this, I helped to develop a francophone branch of Upstream, which is how En Amont came to be.

CPD: In your opinion, what are the most important social determinants of health on which Canada needs to act?

SPL: I see that question on two axes: available income and education. Many people are seeing their real income decrease. Some people describe this as the crumbling of the middle class, but we also need to think of those who are even lower on the salary ladder, for whom a lowering of the minimum income could be catastrophic.

As well, the question of public services is very important to me. If we privatize, people will have to pay for services directly. The mode of payment is no longer progressive, as it is for purely public services sustained through taxes. This lowering of public services is a drain on people's disposable income and increases inequalities. I'm the first to say ·that the current system in Quebec has its weaknesses, but there are ways of innovating within the public system to make it more effective. We need to find ways of reinvesting where it is most efficient, and that means at the front line, in primary care.

CPD: And to reinvest in primary care, where do we start? What are the concrete steps to see clear results?

SPL: We need to make outpatient care more effective - for example, permitting family doctors to have multidisciplinary teams that include nurses, and giving them greater access to labs and medical imaging so that patients are more satisfied.

CPD: With that, how do we attract health professionals to primary care? Are we talking regional premiums, or something else?

SPL: The majority of doctors understand that we are already very well paid, and that we can't really ask for more. Above all, we need to improve the practice environment so that the work of doctors is more convenient, more efficient. Doctors need the tools that will make them happy with the services they offer and patients happy with the services they receive. There is also the question of the social determinants of health, putting the questions of where we need to act upstream at the centre. When I was in Yellowknife, I frequently saw the same patient in emergency. The patient frequently called the ambulance for chest pain, but really what he needed was a meal and a place to rest. I often thought it would cost a lot less if we could secure him housing, three meals a day, and social supports than it would to pay for regular $400 ambulance trips and the price of a consult and lab tests in emergency.

CPD: How can we integrate politics into our practice without necessarily being elected or a party member? What can a doctor do to be able to say they are politically active?

SPL: First you have to follow the news, inform yourself, debate. We have to become aware of the social determinants of health. And you have to take a position, become part of a movement.

When I did my campaign, I met many people who were afraid that if I was elected, we would lose a doctor. I explained that I was limited in what I could do in my role as a doctor and that politics was a way to have a much larger impact on their health, by advocating for decent housing, affordable medications, etc. That's what will really change the lives of my patients.

CPD: How can we encourage our colleagues – other doctors and students – to be interested in this process?

SPL: Medicine is much more engaged that it was in earlier decades. We see this in the development of new university departments. Social medicine has become integrated into the academic sphere. The next step is to transform these ideas into public policy, through advocacy, through collective mobilization, through meetings with political figures.

CPD: For you, what are the major current health concerns for the country?

SPL: Definitely privatization of healthcare and access to primary care. For example, we need more neighbourhood clinics, more care delivered by other health professionals, and to not be oriented toward specialist care any more than necessary. These elements are fundamental and linked: the better the access, the less people will be tempted toward private care as a solution. They also link to one of the values shared by Canadians from one ocean to another: Medicare and the Canada Health Act.

CPD: Are there people who have inspired your journey?

SPL: There are many. Recently I read the biography of Robert Cliche, a Quebec lawyer and judge who was leader of the Quebec wing of the New Democratic Party in the 1960s. I'm also inspired by people like Tommy Douglas and others who have been active for the NDP; it's my political family.

CPD: What impact would you like to leave as a politically engaged doctor?

SPL: I hope to be part of a political movement that reduces inequalities. We saw it in 2012 in Quebec; it's something that is latent, as if the public was waiting for a movement to emerge. I want to be part of that and contribute as I can.

CPD: What is the best advice that you received during your training?

SPL: During my residency in British Columbia, my boss, Dr Steve Beerman, always said to me, "It's a humble profession." He wanted us to understand that even though we were doctors, we had very little power, but that we should work to improve things without taking all the weight on our shoulders.

French version available at - http://hdl.handle.net/2429/60457

▎▎ Chapter 11 ▎▎

Habitat: Considering the Bigger Picture of Our Patients' Lives

Murray Lee (Family Doctor) – Kimberly Williams

Health is impacted by so many factors, of which the healthcare system is just a small part. Ideas about the impact of the environment on human health drove Dr Murray Lee to create his company, Habitat Health Impact Consulting, which strives to "help people understand how changes to social, economic and physical environment can affect humans." The environment constantly changes, and Habitat works with organizations to mitigate the negative impacts on health as these changes occur. Dr Lee is a visionary who is not afraid to challenge the next generation of medical students to truly understand the complexities of the healthcare system. He also teaches them to understand the limitations of physicians to improve the lives of patients unless we are willing to try and change the external factors affecting their health. Since graduating from medical school, Dr Lee has been a champion for primary care, working as a family physician in rural Alberta and now in Naujaat, Nunavut.

Some of the work that Habitat has done includes undertaking a community health effects assessment of a liquid natural gas facility in northern British Columbia. The Habitat team interviewed over fifty stakeholders in key organizations as well as in First Nations communities to better understand potential effects on infectious disease transmission, mental well-being, public safety, diet and nutrition, socioeconomic health effects, and Aboriginal health. Their work in various communities monitors health indicators to ensure that the facility is not having a negative impact on local communities.

Dr Lee has a large impact in educating medical students at the University of Calgary through its population health course. In the past five years, he has dramatically changed the curriculum in order to get medical students out into the community to really see the impacts of socio-economic factors on patients. He is not afraid to push medical students on ideas such as "meeting patients where they are at."

As a medical student and now resident physician, I have been inspired by Dr Lee's ability to ask hard questions, to challenge traditional ideas about health, and to not be afraid to remind future physicians of the political side of medicine. As a mentor, he supported the medical student–driven creation of a global health concentration at the University of Calgary, devoting time and effort to a program to ensure a social justice perspective was always present. As a friend, he has taught me not to accept that change cannot happen. He has reminded me that, as a medical student and now resident, I have the ability to try and change the system to be more equitable. In November of 2015, I sat down with Dr Lee to discuss medical education, Aboriginal health, and the complexities of the healthcare environment.

▮▮ Kimberly Williams: You were the physician in medical school who reminded me that trust was the key not only to understanding our patients, but to treating them. In my first week of medical school, you told us that a patient decides in the first thirty seconds whether they trust us or not. If patients do not trust us, they are not going to tell us what we need to know in order to effectively treat them. You also taught me that trust is something that society gives physicians. However, with this trust comes the responsibility to not just impact the life of the patient in front of me, but to work to ensure the health of society. If I want to help ensure healthy societies, I need to look outside the hospital at the factors impacting the health of my individual patients. What are the biggest forces impacting your patients currently?

■■ **Murray Lee:** There are many forces that shape the lives of my patients in Naujaat, Nunavut. The two biggest forces affecting them right now are colonization and housing. The Inuit, compared to other populations, have a culture in tremendous flux. There are proximal changes occurring that have a direct impact on my patients' health, which include language, food, education, and many other social determinants of health.

In regard to managing these proximal factors, housing is a simple and practical determinant that, if improved, would drastically impact the health of this population. In Naujaat, 50 per cent of the population is under the age of eighteen, and the average age of having your first child is eighteen years. Hence, there is an ongoing additive baby boom. There are huge numbers of children having children. Houses are not built fast enough. It will only continue to get worse. There needs to be improved planning around this issue to ensure that members of the community have access to housing in order to optimize their health.

You also need to change external forces in order to influence health, especially colonization. So much of decolonization is about improving a lack of control. To take a paternalistic view and take more control away from this vulnerable population by saying they are sick – especially when they do not think they are sick – is wrong. At the community level, a lot of the pathology comes from this control and actually causes adverse medical outcomes. For someone to come in as a result of a culture that has lost control, to then scold them for not having control over their lives is wrong. Telling patients, "I can fix this, you need me, and you will disappoint me gravely if you do not" is just perpetuating the power dynamic that is already negatively impacting their health.

We need to meet populations where they are at instead of prescribing our own expectations on them. In populations where people have a lot to deal with, my solution is to have them define their own illness and then let them tell me when they want my help. I try to do it in a culturally appropriate way, with a light touch.

■■ **KW:** You have an interest in the social determinants of health. On a personal level, why does that matter to you?

■■ **ML:** I have found that medicine as I was trained to do it was not hugely creative or effective. It may have been the lack of creativity that drew me away from it and toward the social determinants of health. I was interested in culture, place, and how health would play out in specific contexts. I came late to this understanding of health because it was never taught to me in medical school.

I did a lot of travelling as a rural family doctor early in my practice. At that time, I realized that I had a core set of skills in a context that had a large variability in health and the experience of health. Socrates once said, "The disease is cultural to the place." I really believe that, because I started to recognize these other patterns and causes of ill health that were outside the core skills that I had. I could only address a small, core part of the problem. My approach now is to recognize the limitations that I have and not overstep my ability.

I also try not to interfere in my patients' lives. It has been said that physicians "cure sometimes, treat often, and comfort always." I believe that is what clinical medicine really does. It's a caring profession; physicians are good at helping the sick. But clinical medicine doesn't do much to impact the population in general. I hugely admire people who advocate and make change in a community at large. I have definitely not mastered that. My biggest struggle at work is in stepping away from my limited role as a clinician helping those who know they're suffering and looking for ways to address the upstream causes in the community as a whole.

KW: If you don't feel like you addressed the social determinants of health appropriately in your clinical work, how else have you tried to do that within your career?

ML: I started to do this nearly ten years ago by developing a career in the application of health impact assessment to address the social determinants of health. At that time, I co-created the company Habitat Health Impact Consulting. It works to look at a change that is about to happen and assess how this will impact health. Our company has been central in building practice standards in this area, and Habitat is a well-known leader in this area.

KW: You have long been involved in undergraduate medical teaching. Why do you enjoy working with medical students?

ML: There are people in every class who have the skills to make an impact on the societal level; they are well ahead of what I could teach them. It is hard because I am tasked to teach the bulk of medical students anyway. I almost feel like it is the university's job to not squander that. If we make those who have broader skills just into clinicians, then we squander their potential. One of my roles might be to lean on the medical school so that we do not do that.

KW: What medical students are taught is so imperative to the type of clinician they will become, not just the medical knowledge but the rest of their skills. Do you have any recent experiences of when students are highly aware of the context of the patient?

ML: Recently I was teaching a communications session to medical students in their first few months of school. This was a small-group session where I had a very eloquent student who was struggling while interviewing a patient. I pulled the student out of the interview room to try and figure out why she was struggling. What was enlightening was that she was not struggling because she did not want to get to know this patient better or did not know what questions to ask or lacked a sense of curiosity, but because she was concerned about going to an intimate place for a patient without having the ability to help them. I sometimes also have this fear. It was not only the context of the patient's life, but also the context of the interview that she was acutely aware of.

KW: Our understanding of the social determinants of health is very much fortified by patient contact. Can you think of an individual story that helps illuminate these concepts?

ML: A few years ago I was in Nunavut with a medical student and we were called to the home of Leo, a local man who had fallen off the radar for a couple of days. The RCMP had been called to the house to check on him and when they entered, a single shot had been fired. We were called in to provide medical support.

What the medical student and I saw was like an episode of *CSI*. Leo had fallen forward, face first, onto an open bible. There was blood everywhere around his head, probably three to four liters. Montréal Canadiens paraphernalia was all around and, I remember, a Stephen Harper election ad was playing on his television. A 22-caliber rifle was lying on the floor next to him. That memory is ingrained in my mind; the sight, the smell, the sadness. He had been there for three days by himself thinking about suicide before pulling the trigger when the RCMP arrived. This is maybe what causes me the most pain: his isolation – socially, geographically, and culturally.

The *Globe and Mail* was doing a long series on Nunavut at that time. They had spent some time with Leo and wrote about his life because they felt he was emblematic of what has gone on in the North. Leo went to a residential school, experienced abuse, used recreational drugs, and had been a drug dealer for some time. Ironically, the *Globe and Mail* special came out the week Leo shot himself. On our way the funeral that Saturday, I quickly swung by my clinic and saw a picture of Leo on my computer screen. He was on the cover of the *Globe and Mail*. They broke the Nunavut feature the day of his funeral, just three days after his death, without any idea that he had died.

The photographer for the story who had come to meet Leo, on his blog, talked about how much Leo's death stuck with him. He called Leo's death "yet another senseless tragedy." I agree his story was tragic and the context rich, but when you think about all the things that led Leo to end his life, I do not know if it was senseless. There are predictable patterns that were not about him. He was a man who grew up in the wrong place at the wrong time. He experienced all this hardship, which was channelled through his being because of where he was from and when he was born. Someone 1,000 km south would have had a different outcome, as would an Inuk born a generation before or a generation after. On an individual level I believe the social determinants of health are really just circumstance, unlike at the population level where they can be changed. To me, Leo's death seemed somewhat inevitable based on the external factors impacting his life.

The part I find hard with suicide is not the death, but the days of utter despair in a life where someone has probably thought about suicide for a long time. I find the level of psychic angst and despair that someone in this situation goes through unimaginable. It is so unbelievably unfair. I tell this story to my students, because it is still hard for me to remember, but it reminds me of the bigger picture of our patients' lives.

KW: Who is it that you most admire? Is there a role model who has inspired your approach to this work?

ML: I have a lot of role models: the classic rural family physicians that are committed to a community, who bring skills and empathy every day to their work. Dr Hal Irving is a rural Alberta family physician. In his town they used to plough a path from his front door to the hospital because he was always available. He had rock-solid skills, was well informed, and knew what in his community he could or couldn't impact.

KW: How do you look upstream in your work?

ML: I continuously look for role models. I am always looking for the people who are able to do clinical practice, reflect upon the upstream challenges, and then make an impact on the population level. I am on the lookout for anyone doing that work because I do not feel like I have succeeded in that challenge.

My biggest fear working up north is that my commitment to a community has created an opportunity cost to my patients. I try not to do harm. I tell myself I am doing good work because I am competent and not creating conflict, and that I am protecting them from what I don't like, such as polypharmacy or forced agency. Yet I wonder: Would someone else be there who could establish a traditional food bank or build houses and make a greater change?

KW: What type of political culture do you believe would improve health outcomes?

ML: That political culture would produce good health outcomes by being caring and not blaming people for circumstances beyond their control. It would foster independence and autonomy while recognizing inequity. The political system would try to fix things, without undercutting autonomy and freedom, making it both libertarian and socialist. It is important not to interfere with agency and independence. If someone wants to live a full life with less health, we need to tolerate that. Ultimately, I believe the system should focus on fixing the societal level without interfering with the individual.

▪▪ Chapter 12 ▪▪

Rejecting Indifference in the Face of Death

Joanne Liu (Médecins Sans Frontières/Doctors Without Borders) – Claudel Pétrin-Desrosiers

Every single day, Médecins Sans Frontières (MSF)/Doctors Without Borders is at the front lines of epidemics, international humanitarian crises, civil conflicts, and wars. They treat without prejudice; they act for human dignity. At the head of this Nobel Prize–winning organization sits Dr Joanne Liu, a Canadian pediatrician who usually works at Sainte-Justine Hospital in Montreal. These days, as international president of MSF, she she travels around the world to visit MSF camps, to provide healthcare where there is none, and to bring relief to thousands of people.

Dr Liu has gained international fame in the past few months, as the organization she is leading has been one of the very few to quickly and successfully react to the Ebola outbreak in West Africa. Furthermore, MSF is still operating in Syria, and has been extremely active on the Mediterranean Sea in the midst of the refugee crisis. Involved with MSF for more than twenty years, Dr Liu has made it her personal motto to always keep the interests of her patients at the top of her priorities. Before making any decision, she asks herself, "How will that change the lives of my patients?" Her first mission is to bring relief and not get lost in all the bureaucracy.

Extremely down to earth, Dr Liu is an inspiring physician who strives to break the wall of apathy toward death and conflicts. She reminds us daily that, as doctors, we have a powerful role to play in society. We can't stay silent when we see injustices, and we must keep our patients at the centre of our actions.

■■ **Claudel Pétrin-Desrosiers:** What drove you to study medicine? Could you speak to me of any striking moments in your journey?

■■ **Joanne Liu:** What I remember most is in my adolescence, I was on a great quest to find the raison d'être, a sort of existential quest. I did a lot of reading, and read a lot of books in that period about these questions. I read several books on spirituality, the great classics and some more documentary books like Camus's *The Plague*. That's a big book for me, because it relates to a doctor's battle against a disease that he doesn't have the tools to fight. What comes out in the book is the humanity of the doctor, his will to accompany his patients on their journeys. One passage in particular struck me, when the doctor is asked the question, "What drives you to continue, even though you see clearly all of these people around you who die of the plague?" and he responds, "I never got used to death." That struck me, because I'd always thought it indecent to make death banal, that it is indecent to get used to it. I really liked two other books, one being *Et la paix, docteur?*, which shares the journey of a physician around the world with MSF, as he does his best despite war. The other was on the eradication of smallpox, which I find extraordinary because smallpox is an awful disease that no longer exists in Canada because of the leadership of the people who fought to eradicate it. I would say that these three books, above all, gave me beautiful models of doctors with a social vocation, when instead around me I mostly had an image of the doctors with the biggest houses in town.

At seventeen, I left for Katimavik, and later for Canadian Crossroads International. I'd always believed in communal life and in sharing. I spent three months in Mali in West Africa. There I saw the standard of living people had, and that's when it clicked. I decided I'd go into medicine to go work in developing countries. From that moment on, all of my choices in my studies and my professional life were made with these objectives. I did everything to have a specialty that was exportable, that would be needed where I wanted to go. This brought me to pediatrics, as I'd heard it said that in developing countries over half of the patients seen were children. I also wanted to be in emergency, on the front lines, to be where there's no one else. I also wanted to have the tools to be useful, to not be an encumbrance. That's why I did my specialty in pediatric emergency medicine in New York. I chose New York in order to be exposed to something outside Canada, and above all, to be exposed to bullet wounds and stabbings.

CPD: At the end of your residency, what brought you to MSF?

JL: I always wanted to go on a mission with MSF. When I did my residency in the United States, it was in 1994, the same time as the genocide in Rwanda. I got involved as a volunteer in the MSF offices. I was torn because I still couldn't be on the ground to lend a hand. I spoke to the doctors; I screened the files. MSF embodied my values: people who are on the ground, who take risks, who will use their voice to speak in the name of those without voice. I wanted to go beyond the clinical, to be able to denounce injustices. At that level, MSF corresponded exactly to my personality.

CPD: The need to speak in the name of those with no voice, to be able to denounce injustice, it's not everyone who feels the need to do that. Where does that come from for you?

JL: I've always had quite strong opinions. It's anchored in my

133

personality since I was very little. I don't necessarily describe myself as an activist, I don't go out in the streets protesting, but I want to be able to set a limit, to say no loud and strong, to say, "That's enough, the line has been crossed." I wanted to have the tools to do that, and I found them with MSF.

CPD: We speak more and more about women in decision-making roles. How can we favour female leadership?

JL: That's never really been a big question in my life; I always charged right in wherever I wanted to. When I got into medicine, there was already more balance – we were nearly preferred. In terms of feminization, that's a very interesting question. One part is socialization; one part is genetic baggage. I often ask myself the question today, but I think that growing up as a visible minority in Quebec City was more difficult than being a woman. It was a much bigger obstacle being Chinese and being raised in the sixties and seventies in Quebec, which was at the time completely white.

CPD: Did that perspective from when you were young change your practice and your outlook on difference? We know that it's often the people who are most different, the most vulnerable, that suffer the most health inequalities.

JL: This question of difference is a reality I lived every day when I was young. In some ways, what was clearest in my life was my difference. We know that children can be cruel, so I had to build a shell. I always wanted to show leadership, for example. I told myself one thing: I wanted to be smarter than all of those kids; I wanted to succeed in beating them. It's a pretty frequent phenomenon. I became the best at everything: in sports, math, French, even in religion, although I didn't take the religion classes. The point is, difference makes a mark; it fashions you as a person. We are left with two choices: accept the difference and rise above, or be overwhelmed and fall below. When I got to McGill, I immersed myself in a Chinese scene. Even my roommate was Chinese. She did her masters in sociology on the first generation of Chinese born in Canada and their high level of performance. Her conclusion was that we performed well because of our difference. There was an enormous amount of pressure on the first generation born in the country, even more because of the enormous sacrifices their parents had made to get established.

CPD: What motivates you day after day? How do you keep up your energy, despite all the difficult geopolitical situations in which MSF intervenes?

JL: Whether it's as a doctor on the ground in the Democratic Republic of the Congo, as the person in charge of a needs-assessment mission, or as international president of MSF, the important thing is to always keep the patient in mind. The primary objective is treating people. I see all my choices that way. Before doing anything, to participate in projects, to speak on the public stage, I always ask myself the question, "How is what I'm doing right now going to change the lives of patients? Does it add to the social mission of MSF, which is to bring medical support to people in need?" If I don't see that link, from near or far, I question the decision. That's what motivates me. I refuse to be a bureaucrat, to lose the thread of the primary mission of bringing care to patients.

CPD: I imagine that you see changes at the local level when you bring care. Does that act as positive reinforcement?

JL: Of course. We're extremely privileged when we do emergency medicine. The impact of our actions is enormous. For example, in Kunduz, in the last year, we treated more than 20,000 people and did more than 5,000 orthopedic surgeries and traumas. It's clear that we make a big difference for our patients. But by our testimony, we can shine the light on the actions necessary for long-term change.

CPD: For you, what are the greatest health challenges in Canada and around the world?

JL: For me, it's access to care, in Canada and elsewhere in the world. Even in Quebec, there are 40,000 people without access to a family doctor, who find themselves going to walk-in clinics without receiving continuity of care, who don't have a patient-provider relationship. At the end of the line, it's patching people up, or what I call McMedicine. It's not good enough. We also see it with an ageing population, which will pose many challenges to the country with a flagrant lack of home care. We have to re-humanize our care, and make care accessible for the elderly, the disabled, and people with reduced mobility. There is a lot to fix. In Canada, we often try to have everything at once, but we have to make choices and establish priorities. At the moment, we favour short-term gain, based on political power, rather than real needs. We need reflective leadership, leadership ready to make real choices.

At the international level, access to care is a real problem, especially in situations of armed conflict. What is happening today in Afghanistan, where our hospital has been bombed numerous times, is an example of the problem. We had to close our centre: more than a million Afghans no longer have access to the trauma care that we've been offering for four years. We see the same thing in Yemen. The country is in a state of total war, where everything is targeted, including health centres. There are also the problems of healthcare deserts. For example, in the

Congo or the Central African Republic there are total healthcare deserts where people can walk for three weeks before arriving at the first clinic. With the phenomena of migration, wars, and economic and climatic problems that we see now, we will find ourselves with populations that are impoverished, unemployed, vulnerable, and with a very precarious access to care.

CPD: What role do you think doctors have in society?

JL: For me, a doctor, like anyone else, has to understand that they have a social responsibility in a global sense. They must play their role as a doctor, but also as a citizen of the world. If not, it just doesn't work. This question of social responsibility is also very intimate, different for each of us, but for doctors many of the elements of this response are in the Hippocratic Oath taken at the beginning of training. Medicine today is more than a social status; it's a social responsibility.

CPD: What footprint would you like to leave as a pediatric emergency doctor and as president of MSF?

JL: I'd like to do my best to accomplish the tasks with which I've been entrusted. I'd like to break down the wall of indifference to the suffering of the world, the coolness in the face of death and violence. I find the dehumanization of armed conflicts, of phenomena like the refugee crisis, completely indecent. We protect ourselves because it's the best way not to have to do something, to stay as nothing but spectators. I fight this indifference through healthcare.

CPD: Tell me about role models that have influenced your journey, that have pushed you to do more.

JL: There's a Buddhist monk, Thich Nhat Than, who during

137

the Vietnam War created something called Engaged Buddhism. It's the idea of having an engagement outside of prayer, to translate our spirituality into concrete acts. During the entire Vietnam War, he brought people aid. He incarnated Buddhist values through everyday actions. That's someone I find very inspiring, because he also speaks of full consciousness, of the significance of the actions we take, of non-violence. I'm also part of a generation that couldn't help but be inspired by Gandhi. He was a great person. What he was able to achieve through non-violence is extremely remarkable. The struggle of Nelson Mandela is also very impressive. These are three people who pursued their struggle through non-violence and were able to achieve their objectives. It's a longer road, but it's probably non-violence that gave them their lasting power. I believe that violence doesn't bring sustainable solutions. It may bring ephemeral gains, but they are not built to last.

CPD: What is the best advice you received during your training?

JL: I remember when I did my masters, my supervisor told me, "It's great that you have this post with MSF. You're in a state of 'nothing to lose.' You're there for the patients, not for your career. Continue to keep their interests above your personal interests." He also told me to avoid taking things personally. Being the head of MSF International comes with a lot of exposure; it's normal to take a few hits. It's the price to pay, but you can't lose sight of your primary goal: the patients. This supervisor also told me, "Losing personal capital for our patients, it's a small price to pay." The struggle I'm in is for them, not for me.

French version available at - http://hdl.handle.net/2429/60457

◼◼ Chapter 13 ◼◼

On Motivation, Mentors, and Medicare

Danielle Martin (Canadian Doctors for Medicare) – Vivian Tam

There are few plans to transform our healthcare system as clear as Dr Danielle Martin's. A formidable visionary, she has championed efforts to enhance Canadian Medicare since her graduation from medical school. In her first year of practice as a family physician, she co-founded Canadian Doctors for Medicare (CDM), an advocacy group dedicated to preserving and optimizing publicly funded healthcare. Since its inception, physicians involved with CDM have become recognized champions of healthcare reform, provoking widespread discussion across medical schools and major media outlets regarding improvement and innovation in medicare.

Recently, Dr Martin pitched three "Big Ideas" to further enhance our healthcare system: universal coverage of prescription medications; improved stewardship of medical tests and interventions; and a basic income guarantee for vulnerable Canadians. She says these ideas will enhance medicare by making health more accessible and the healthcare system more sustainable – and I, like many others, believe her. As vice president of Medical Affairs and Health Systems Solutions at Women's College Hospital in Toronto, Dr Martin is working at the forefront of healthcare innovation. She has a vision honed through years of policy work and clinical practice, including within some of Ontario's most vulnerable communities. She is convinced that improving the accessibility of medicare will mitigate the impact of other social barriers to health, and with her demonstrated talent and conviction, the conversations she has started will doubtless reverberate to improve the health of all Canadians.

As a medical student, I've long since realized that I too want to use my career to pursue health equity and social justice, and Dr Martin is the compellingly articulate visionary whose work I aspire to emulate. Of this, I can say with certainty that I am not alone. In September of 2015, I was honoured to sit down with Dr Martin to discuss her motivations, Canada's political culture, and what it means to her to advocate for health systems change as a physician.

■■ Vivian Tam: How has working with your patients shaped your understanding of the way that upstream factors like income, housing, and food security affect people's health?

■■ Danielle Martin: For all healthcare workers and physicians, the upstream determinants are where we bump up against the limits of our own training. If we're honest, most of us experience the importance of the social determinants of health when we experience frustration about our own inability to help our patients stay healthy or get well, because there are some things for which our medical tools are not useful. So we mostly experience it as frustration, and for many of us that can become a driving force in the work that we do.

■■ VT: How has that frustration fuelled your work, as a health advocate, clinician, and educator?

■■ DM: Most of my work has been in the area of healthcare systems, as opposed to the social determinants, but we know that equitable access to healthcare is a determinant of health. It probably determines about 25 per cent of health. My view is that, although the social determinants are incredibly important and require our collective advocacy, one of the things that can help to equalize inequities in the social determinants is a strong, equitable, publicly funded healthcare system. A publicly funded healthcare system serves as a redistributive tool in a community or society where access to the social determinants is inequitable and imperfect. As long as we have an inequitable set of social determinants, we will need to rely in part on a strong, publicly funded healthcare system to provide a cushion for people.

■■ **VT:** You've previously proposed three big ideas to transform the healthcare system: a universal pharmacare system, choosing medical interventions wisely, and a basic income guarantee. How did you arrive at these three targets in particular, and what has progress been like since you first proposed them?

■■ **DM:** The three ideas have now evolved into six ideas, and I'm writing a book about them. These things evolve over time. For starters, none of these are my ideas. They are not concepts that I came up with; they are my "picks" as I scan the policy landscape for the concepts that I think would have a big impact on the health of Canadians and are within the realm of the achievable in the short-to-medium term. Any given advocate will likely name different targets, so these may not necessarily be the best or most important, but they're the ones that I'm most engaged with and where I think the biggest impact is to be had.

The first relates to the implementation of universal pharmacare in Canada, or the notion that we should be bringing prescription medicine under medicare, and I think we are seeing quite a lot of movement on that file right now. Where it will land, I don't know. The growing numbers of healthcare providers and physicians in particular who have been active on this file have helped to bring the issue into the public eye, and I'm thrilled to see that.

Improving stewardship is a notion that has been gaining traction in the Canadian medical community through the Choosing Wisely Campaign, and I know that medical students are becoming leaders in this conversation. Patients and citizens, as well as healthcare providers, need to work to reorient our system to ensure that the tests, treatments, and interventions we use are actually likely to improve health. After all, that's the purpose of a healthcare system. If we can do better in this regard, not only will the quality of care improve, our system will be more sustainable.

Basic income is not a new idea; we all know what an important determinant of health poverty is, and many more impressive advocates than I have advocated for it. What I like about the basic income concept is that it is both a realistic and achievable solution to poverty in Canada, and it is a means of raising the conversation about the determinants of health and the importance of income to the health of Canadians. It seems to be under discussion: we've heard provincial politicians from quite a few provinces talk about running pilot projects, and mayors from a number of different communities across the country have raised the possibility as well, so we may yet see a basic income pilot taking place in Canada in the next year or two.

VT: How does your interest in healthcare transformation speak to you on a personal level?

DM: I grew up in a family of people committed to social justice who were very involved in activism and politics, both the "small-p" kind and the "big-P" kind. So I have always assumed that, no matter what I was doing in my life and career, I would be involved in advocacy work of some kind around issues of social justice. That's a core part of who I am and what I need to do in order to feel that I'm of use in the world.

▌█ VT: I decided to go into medicine because I recognized how much privilege I had. My parents were new immigrants to Canada, but my brother and I were very fortunate to grow up in a household where we never wanted for anything. It made me recognize the amount of privilege that goes into being able to say that, and I wanted to advocate for social justice and health equity so that others around me could achieve their potential and lead full and healthy lives, as I have. What drew you to medicine, and what were other career options that you considered?

▌█ DM: I came to medicine late in my development. I did my training in the basic sciences, like many in healthcare. When I graduated, I went to work in politics. I was working in the office of the Liberal health critic under the Harris government in Ontario. That was what awakened my interest in healthcare policy, and it became clear to me that I was committed to a career in it. I came to medicine thinking that I would be most effective and useful in a healthcare policy career if I understood what actually works, and what doesn't, on the ground. So I was not initially driven to medicine by a desire to help individual people; I was driven to medicine by the desire to improve the healthcare system, and I wanted to understand that system from the ground up. That's what led me to medical school, and when I went to medical school I fell in love with family medicine and became much more interested in the one-on-one, longitudinal relationship-based encounters that can also make a difference in the health of individuals, if not in the health of populations. Many people start out with the passion for helping individuals and then are awakened to the possibility of doing something on the system level; in my case, it was the reverse.

▌█ VT: Do you currently practise in rural or remote parts of Ontario?

DM: Not anymore, although I did at the beginning of my career. When I graduated in 2005, I spent about six months working in rural Northern Ontario in a variety of different communities as a locum physician. When I took my current job at the Women's College Hospital as a family doctor, I continued to travel up north on a periodic basis for another three years after that, mostly to one community in northwestern Ontario called Geraldton. I stopped doing that when I had my daughter because it was difficult to manage the travel with a baby. But I do miss it, and it certainly did shape my views a lot on what works and doesn't work in healthcare reform and the needs of more rural and remote communities.

VT: Is there any particular reason why you wanted to start your career working in a remote or rural part of Ontario?

DM: I just felt that that was where the need was. When I was a medical student, I went to Sioux Lookout in Northern Ontario, which is a community that serves a large number of First Nations communities in the North, and I was very affected by that experience. My brief time spent on reserve there was very formative in terms of helping me understand the deep injustices and inequities that exist and that First Nations peoples in Canada have to overcome in order to achieve health. After that experience, I promised myself I would go back and make what contributions I could as a clinician, which are small in the face of broader issues at hand but still need to be addressed.

VT: Is there a particular patient or story from that period that left an impact on you?

DM: When I was working in Sioux Lookout as a brand new, just-graduated family doctor – this would have been in the fall of 2005 – an eleven-year-old child was flown down to the emergency department I was working in from one of the remote fly-in reserves, having unsuccessfully tried to hang herself for the second time. I just realized that there was no medicine for that despair. The issues in that community and for that little girl ran so deep and were so intergenerational that as a healthcare provider there was so little that I could do once I made sure she hadn't broken her neck. I was very affected by that.

VT: One of my favourite quotes is by Rudolf Virchow, who said, "Politics is nothing but medicine on a grander scale." How would you reflect on this?

DM: Health is a fundamentally political concept, so I agree with that. If you think about the social determinants in the broadest sense, every policy in government is a health policy, and every ministry in government is a ministry of health. What's decided and what's done in education, social services, transportation, or the environment, all eventually have a major impact on health. And so, given how highly Canadians rate their health and the heath of their families as priorities in every public poll, I think it's helpful to understand that when we talk about the importance of health, we're not only talking about the importance of healthcare but, in fact, we're talking about the importance of health in all policies.

VT: And do you think that this is true only in Canada, or is it a global commonality?

DM: It's absolutely global. If you improve people's economic situation, if you educate the girls in a community, or provide people with access to tools of self-determination, their health improves. The question of whether you frame those interventions as health interventions, economic development interventions, or social justice tools, ultimately, when you make the world a fairer and better place, you also improve the health of the community.

VT: Do you think it has taken longer for Canada to get to that realization, or is this just the natural course in our evolution as a country?

DM: I don't think Canada has made that realization as a country. People tend to place healthcare policies and other policies in opposition to each other, as though there is tension between them. I think we "know" this from the literature, or we can say intellectually that it's true, but in practice, in our political culture we tend to behave as though there is a choice to be made between health or healthcare and other things. I reject this paradigm, but I don't think we're living in an enlightened age on that front; there's much work that still needs to be done.

VT: What changes do you think need to be made in our political culture for us to make this realization, and to act on it?

DM: Unfortunately, the political rhetoric around the healthcare budget crowding out other expenditures in the province has been really damaging. Budgetary decisions made by governments across the country to talk about improving population health via, for example, hiring more doctors or nurses at the same time that they're cutting social assistance rates, reinforces the false tension between healthcare and all other social policies. How do you change a political culture or narrative? In part, I think that advocacy groups and groups of healthcare providers can help to burst those bubbles, but we also need courageous political leaders who are willing to reframe those conversations. Unfortunately, I think that particular kind of leadership has been in short supply.

VT: You've been asked to join a number of political parties at different levels of government, and many would say that the political arena is where decisions to transform healthcare can be made. Would you ever consider journeying into politics?

DM: No, I would not. I would put a small caveat on that by saying, if I were to have reason to believe that the only way I could be effective in making change and improving the system for my community was to go into politics, then I suppose I would have to consider it. I count myself lucky that I don't feel that way. I feel that there are lots of good ways that I can make a contribution and help to contribute to change. Actually, in some ways I can be more effective where I am, relatively unconstrained in my capacity to express my views and to push political leaders to do what I think needs to be done, than I would be if I chose to enter politics myself. So I suppose one should never say never, but I'm not tempted.

VT: What do you think is the biggest barrier to healthcare transformation?

DM: Maybe the biggest barrier to healthcare transformation is that we keep talking about barriers. Sometimes I think we're trapped in a negative narrative in the Canadian healthcare system that doesn't do justice to what's good about what we've built and what's worth building upon, and the tremendous opportunities available to us. You talked about privilege, and how privileged we are, those of us who have meaningful work that we can do that contributes to the betterment of our communities. We've got hundreds of thousands of people going to work every day across our healthcare system who want to do the right thing, and whose energy can be channelled and capitalized upon to make things better. One of my goals right now is to shift us to a positive conversation about the good things we could be doing – hence the "Big Ideas" narrative – instead of dwelling on what's not working. What would you say is the biggest barrier?

VT: Politics, because I feel like we have a lot of the solutions we need and a lot of the evidence to back up the solutions we propose. But in order to actualize them, you need political will. If our different levels of government committed to, for example, implementing pharmacare, then it could be done a lot more quickly.

DM: I agree. People talk about political will, and of course we need it, but I think the pointy end of political will is courage. Political representatives have to get their courage from us. We have to give them the courage to take risks, to go out on a limb, or to try things where some outcomes may be uncertain. So is that the fault of the politicians, or the citizens for not lifting our representatives up on a wave of demand for these solutions? My question and interest is in how you create that wave of demand.

VT: If you could recommend medical learners gain just one skill to be successful health advocates, what would it be?

DM: I would recommend the same skill that I would recommend for being a successful clinician, which is to know yourself. Advocacy is about coalition building, and working together with others who see the world the way you do to try to advance a cause. In order to do that effectively, you need to know what you contribute as an individual, which requires you to have a very clear sense of your own personal strengths, and the areas where you need others to step in and do that work. Every movement needs researchers, evidence synthesis and analysis, communications, a public face, and effective advocacy to government. Every movement needs community building and difficult coalition negotiations. Nobody can do all of those things, so there's no single skill.

What's required is a team of people who are each doing what they do best in harmony with each other. Where intelligent people sometimes fall down is in thinking that their job is to do all of those things. Knowing yourself and what your role is in that is how you can make sure you can be most useful.

VT: You work with individual patients day-to-day, and on a systems level. How do you think one impacts the other?

DM: The two are definitely synergistic. My day-to-day work as a clinician is core to who I am. It allows me to be real in the system-level work that I do: to be realistic about what we can ask of providers in the healthcare system who are working hard and are overloaded; and to understand what's feasible in terms of change and what sounds good on paper but probably wouldn't work in the real world. Vice versa, having an understanding of system-level issues really helps me to help my patients navigate what can be a very complex environment. So the two inform each other. Of course, they also sometimes come into conflict – it's tough to balance, but we all manage.

VT: And certainly not every physician or medical student looks at the systems level as much as you do. What do you think is their responsibility in addressing the social determinants?

DM: Every healthcare provider has a responsibility to be sensitive to and conscious of the social determinants of health, and to incorporate advocacy for their individual patients into their practice. I also think that every healthcare provider has a responsibility to lend their support to initiatives to improve those upstream determinants. That doesn't mean that everybody is going to volunteer hundreds of hours or attend conferences about the social determinants, but each person can contribute in ways acceptable to them. Some people donate money, sign petitions, or sit on a committee. If the goal of the healthcare provider is to improve health for people, then we cannot constrain ourselves to the delivery of healthcare services without trying to understand what it is that actually makes people sick.

VT: Are there any particular books you would recommend that students interested in the upstream factors read?

DM: They should definitely read Ryan Meili's book, *A Healthy Society*, and hopefully my book when it comes out. I also like the books of Atul Gawande; I love his articles in *The New Yorker*, partly because he's such a beautiful writer, but also because he manages to weave the stories of individual patients in with system-level questions and issues in a way that's quite brilliant. For physicians who may not immediately see the link between what they do with the individual and these broader policy questions, he's certainly worth reading. I would also recommend anything written by Don Berwick to students. There was a commencement speech he did for the Harvard Medical School called "To Isaiah" that I still think about. It was another good example of telling the story of an individual patient and linking that to the bigger picture, which is something that is important for medical students to keep front of mind, even when they're busy trying to learn biomedical concepts.

VT: What do you think is the power of individual stories in galvanizing public and political attention to the social determinants of health?

DM: I learned early on in my advocacy career that every issue requires both narrative and evidence. You need both. You can't advocate for something that doesn't have evidence to support it; you need the statistics and to know the numbers and to have those evaluations at your fingertips. But without stories or narrative to put a face to the issue that you're trying to put forward, it never feels real. Humans learn through narrative; you absolutely need stories.

■ Chapter 14 ■

Driven Upstream: The Quest for a Healthy Society

Ryan Meili (Upstream) – Melanie Bechard

Dr Ryan Meili is a family physician with an unwavering passion for the social determinants of health. He currently practises at the Westside Community Clinic in Saskatoon and serves as an assistant professor at the College of Medicine, University of Saskatchewan. Dr Meili is head of the Division of Social Accountability, co-lead of SHARE (Saskatchewan HIV/AIDS Research Endeavour), as well as director of the Making the Links Certificate in Global Health, which provides medical students with first-hand insight into the social determinants through clinical placements in northern Saskatchewan, rural Mozambique, and the SWITCH (Student Wellness Initiative Toward Community Health) inner-city Saskatoon clinic.

A lifelong resident of Saskatchewan, Dr Meili completed his undergraduate studies in human anatomy and languages at the University of Saskatchewan before graduating from the College of Medicine in 2004 and completing residency at the Saskatoon Westwinds Primary Health Centre in 2007. Dr Meili is an active local and global citizen; after an unsuccessful initial application to medical school, he spent five months travelling throughout South America and co-organized the Limbs and Light for Latin America project, which delivered prosthetic limbs to land-mine victims in Nicaragua.

Dr Meili's 2012 book, A Healthy Society: How a Focus on Health can Revive Canadian Democracy, *uses both evidence-based policy and poignant patient stories to propose democratic reforms for a healthier society. Dr Meili continues to advocate for healthy public policy through his roles as vice chair of Canadian Doctors for Medicare, a Broadbent Institute Fellow, Evidence Network expert, and founding director of Upstream: Institute for a Healthy Society.*

As a recently graduated medical student with an interest in health policy and social pediatrics, I have read and admired much of Dr Meili's work from afar. It was exciting to be able to speak with a passionate advocate whose career path I aspire to emulate. I hope the interview below illustrates Dr Meili's inspiring commitment to a healthier society through a focus on the social determinants of health.

Melanie Bechard: Could you start by telling us a little bit more about yourself, both personally and professionally?

Ryan Meili: Sure. I'm a family doctor in Saskatoon. I grew up on a farm in southern Saskatchewan. I completed my medical school and residency here in Saskatoon. Before, during, and after my training, I spent time in other countries: Brazil, Mozambique, India, and the Philippines. Here in Saskatchewan, I've worked in northern regions and pretty much all over rural Saskatchewan. My current practice is in the inner city at the Westside Community Clinic. I am married to Mahli Brindamour, who is a pediatrician, and we have one son, Abraham.

MB: Where do you think your interest in the social determinants of health and health advocacy began?

RM: I came into medical school with an interest in social justice. I was really wanting – with that classic naïveté of medical students and premedical students – to help people and do my part to contribute, and I thought medicine was the most sensible way to do so. You are able to be of direct assistance to people in a pretty meaningful way. My goal was always to work with underserved populations. I remember very clearly at that time thinking about working in low-income countries, and my exposure during medical school changed my thinking a little bit – not away from wanting to work in those areas, but in understanding what really makes a difference and whether we're helping or not. I remember very clearly a lecture where the social determinants of health were introduced to us, and my classmates and me being asked what made the biggest difference in health, and most of the answers being things like genes or culture or access to medical care. Most of us were quite shocked at how much influence money has, how much influence level of education has. It makes sense, but it wasn't where our minds went right away. That struck me and became a bit of a theme to my way of looking at health, connecting some of my political beliefs and interests with my medical practice in a more concrete way.

MB: I had a pretty similar experience in our first-year Determinants of Community Health course here at the University of Toronto. I came to medicine with a background that was both rooted in some social sciences as well as in the biomedical sciences, and I was so glad that there was an area that seemed to marry the two of them and show the connections between the two. It's also a pretty big shocker for people to discover that healthcare is eleventh or twelfth on the list of factors that make the biggest difference, especially when you consider where the greatest proportion of our healthcare dollars go. We're much more focused on acute care rather than the social determinants. You mentioned that you came to medical school with a desire already to help serve underserved populations. Where did this desire come from? Was it shaped by anything that you experienced early on in your life or something that a mentor helped to impart to you?

RM: It's a bit of a long story. But to put it briefly, I was around nineteen or twenty, and I was a little bit lost. I didn't have a very clear path. I had a period of opportunity for reflection in which I read lots of books in philosophy and literature and just had some time to think about what I wanted to do and who and how I wanted to be in the world. Life is relatively short. What are we going to do with the time we have? It seemed to me to make the most sense to try and help those who needed it most. And that's when I thought about what my interests were, talents were, and thought I should try to do medicine, in particular where doctors are few or where needs are great.

I'm also Catholic, so these thoughts are informed by social justice, informed by some of my exposures to liberation theology. Before medical school, I ended up spending some time with a diocesan mission in the Northeast Region of Brazil and was exposed to some approaches to faith and social justice that were inspiring to me and have informed the way that I try to work with communities.

There's a priest from Saskatoon, Father Paquin, who was in Brazil for many years. He always talked about how they weren't there evangelizing people, they were being evangelized and were listening and working with a population. Now it seems like a pretty obvious concept, but at the time I think that many of us would first look at medicine and think we're going to do for people, we're going to help serve them, and show them good ways to be. His mission, his practice – and others that I witnessed there – of living alongside people, listening, and facilitating were very important for me to witness.

MB: It seems as though you really entered medicine with eyes open wide, and that was a very conscious decision for you to do so. At least to some extent, everyone comes with some degree of altruism. Why do you think some physicians are able to build their practice with such a focus on social justice and advocacy, whereas others seem to immerse themselves more in strictly clinical matters and aren't as interested in the big, systemic picture?

RM: I think back to my medical school and the rule of thirds. A third of people there really were more traditional: there to make money, there to have a good career. Then about a third were more thinking about the social-service side of things and the altruism. Then the middle third was a combination of the two, interested in the social side of things, but still focused on some degree of comfort. I'm sure that's not a totally accurate representation, but that's sort of how I saw the medical school breaking down.

But in medicine, you have a reflection of the political spectrum of society, and it's not that surprising that you have some people really taking on a more socially minded, community-focused approach to things, and others taking on a more individualistic focus. That may explain part of it. Different specialties also allow for that more easily. Some of the more general specialties have more in-depth relationship elements. If you're in pediatrics, you spend much more time with the patient, and talking with the patient, and understanding circumstances than perhaps someone in anesthesia might do, just by nature of the service you're providing.

Then there's the overt and hidden curriculum. These concepts are talked about in medical school, and there certainly are people who concentrate on them quite a bit, but clinical always wins. Clinical is always the most valued element of our different competencies or different tricks in our medical bags. We're always judged first on our clinical acumen, and there's a hierarchy where those who do the most direct, clinical procedural work are considered the real doctors.

MB: That hidden curriculum is very poorly hidden at times. You do get the sense, whether it's explicitly stated or not, that we're really encouraged to be researchers, practising in urban areas. Schools are often ranked in terms of their research output, but they don't often give as much regard to the student experience or quality of education. It might be time to maybe start looking at whether or not schools are achieving the goals they've set for their population and whether they're producing socially accountable physicians.

RM: At the University of Saskatchewan, I head up our Division of Social Accountability, and a big part of that role is trying to figure out how we, as a medical school, can better serve the priority needs of our communities, and how that informs the work of the medical school. We call that the CARE model (Clinical service, Advocacy, Research, Education), asking in what ways will the work of the medical school actually improve the health of the populations we're serving. In some ways this seems so obvious, but it isn't actually the lens that is most often used. There's been a lot of progress in that direction in the last decade or so, but there's still a lot of work to do.

MB: I'm curious if you bring these goals and ideas to other medical institutions and what the response is, or even what the response is at your own university and what kind of reaction you have faced.

RM: We've been very well supported at the College of Medicine at the University of Saskatchewan in that there's been investment to establish this division and support core projects, like the Making the Links Certificate in Global Health. This program teaches students about the social determinants of health through service-learning experiences in northern Saskatchewan, at the SWITCH student-run, inner-city clinic in Saskatoon, and then through international experiences in countries like Mozambique or Vietnam. We're seeing a real movement at other schools to go in that direction as well, where they are setting up their own committees or offices of social accountability and also starting global health certificates or concentrations similar to Making the Links. That's really positive to see.

The other side is that it's still very much marginal and not mainstream. Northern Ontario School of Medicine is one exception where it's really well integrated, but I'm not on the ground there, so who knows if there's still some resistance amongst some faculty. Here in Saskatchewan, we've seen great uptake of this at an official level, but it's really difficult work – cultural-change work, time-consuming work – to try and move it out to each department so that every student and every resident has an experience of how to become a socially accountable physician.

MB: In my training, there have been opportunities to experience global health and work actively with the social determinants of health, but as you described, the next step is to integrate this well into our traditional curricula, not just having social justice and social accountability as a side interest.

RM: Yes, as more than just an option if you happen to like it. That isn't always preserved when the rubber hits the road of exams, or career choices, or other sorts of "hard" objectives. One other thing that helps is that service learning and social accountability have been integrated into accreditation standards. Now every student must have a service-learning opportunity, and schools must demonstrate how they are committed to social accountability. So that's another way that we can move this. Unfortunately, we all study to the test, we study to accreditation standards, and so if this is a real value, it needs to be required in that testing and in those standards.

■■ MB: Could you describe the organization Upstream a little bit more – what motivated its creation, and what your role is with Upstream?

■■ RM: Upstream is a non-profit, non-partisan organization with a national focus, though its home base is here in Saskatoon. It's an active part of a larger movement to build a healthier society through evidence-based, people-centred ideas. To break that down, we really are trying to reframe Canadian politics around the concept of health as the primary goal. After all, what is government for if it's not to improve our health and well-being? But that's not how we measure the success of governments: we tend to measure through GDP and other numbers that don't necessarily reflect the quality of our lives. Upstream is about refocusing our goal as being health and recognizing that healthcare is not the way you reach that. It's only one element; you need to be looking at the social determinants of health: income, education, healthy nutrition, the wider environment, employment. These are really the stuff of politics, the stuff of government decisions, and that list of determinants is the road map to a healthier society.

Upstream works with academics and advocates who understand the evidence of what the best options are to understand the social determinants of health, and we work to tell the stories of patients or people living in communities that can highlight the individual impacts of policy changes, good or bad. Through that, we build a community of individuals and organizations who are really looking at things through this lens, using this language to describe current struggles and the most hopeful, evidence-informed options to improve the current situation.

Upstream developed from a number of roots. It came from my own experience being a physician and enjoying the practice of medicine very much, but also being frustrated by the limitations of seeing patients, treating them, and then knowing that they're returning to the circumstances that made them ill. It comes from the frustration of knowing that they or their neighbours will be back because we haven't really dealt with the source of their illness. That frustration drove me to become involved in politics – I ran twice for leader of the New Democrats in Saskatchewan – and also to write a book called *A Healthy Society*. Between the book and the campaign, we built up a group that was really committed to these ideas, decided that there was a need and appetite for this work in Canada, and started Upstream to try and do that political frame-changing over the coming years.

We call it Upstream because of a classic story that you've probably heard. It's the story of kids drowning in the river, of people diving in to save these children, and of kid after kid coming down the river. Eventually somebody says, "Who keeps chucking these kids in the river?" and goes upstream to find out. So it's about trying to think proactively instead of reactively, thinking about how we create the conditions for good health in the long term rather than always responding to illness.

■■ MB: That's the more effective and even more financially responsible method of looking after people's health.

■■ RM: Absolutely, and we make the economic argument at times. For example, we ran a campaign last year where we demonstrated that poverty was costing the Saskatchewan economy $3.8 billion per year. That's 5 per cent of our GDP. We used that information as well as stories of people living in poverty to convince the Saskatchewan government to adopt a poverty-reduction strategy. So it can be helpful to bring in those economic arguments. I'm always a little bit cautious of this approach, however, because part of our current frame is that money is the most important thing, and we want to move away from that. We have to wisely know our numbers but really focus in on the fact that what matters most is the quality of our lives, not economic growth at an aggregate level.

■■ **MB:** It's really interesting to hear about your political involvement. I think that as physicians, we have a unique perspective, and that our active involvement in politics is really one of the most effective ways that we can influence health policy in this country. However, when I speak to some of my friends outside of medicine, they'll sometimes say, "I think it's unfair that physicians, who have invested all this training to become medical experts, are now involved in this completely different field," as though it's a waste of clinical training. Even people outside of medicine seem to prioritize the whole idea of the clinical medical expert who maintains that sole focus. Have you encountered any of that pushback?

■■ **RM:** The first time that I ran, there was a comment like that in the newspaper: "You should stay a doctor. We need more doctors. We have plenty of politicians." We train physicians to improve our health. It's the purpose of the profession. The clinical role is the most common set of tools for doing so. But really, the goal is the same. And if physicians use involvement in politics the way Virchow said, seeing politics as medicine on a larger scale, then it's merely an extension of the work and the training, only with a different set of tools.

■■ **MB:** After starting residency about two-and-a-half months ago, I'm finding that time is really limited, and sometimes we have to make some really difficult decisions. I'm torn between coming home and reading up on the clinical cases I saw during the day versus being politically involved and engaged, for example with the Canadian Federation of Medical Students' national pharmacare campaign. We can be excellent clinicians and we can be excellent advocates, but there are a limited number of hours in the day. How have you found that balance? How have you maintained a successful, useful clinical practice that serves individual patients in front of you, while also maintaining that systems-level perspective?

RM: Residency is a particular period where it's really tough to have those outside interests apart from the clinical, just because the load of learning is so great. It's one of the areas that worries me the most, because we tend to have really keen early medical students, slightly less keen clerks, and then residents disappear from the global health initiatives or student-run clinics. We lose them at a critical period in their lives, where they may or may not come back to that kind of advocacy or socially minded clinical efforts. At the same time, life is long, and there are seasons for everything, and right now, you really need to concentrate on the clinical side of things. You already have some great background in the advocacy, so to shift the balance for a while may be appropriate. I confess I've personally found it to be a challenge. I want to do more of everything because I love the clinical work, I love the political advocacy work, I love the teaching and research. I've now come to place where I feel I have the best of all worlds. I get to do the front-line care and work with patients who really need it. I also get to do some big-picture thinking and acting that reflects what I'm learning from the clinical practice. When you can strike a balance, when you can find the right mix, it's really valuable because it allows you to be informed in your advocacy by the real lives of patients and informed in your clinical care by the social determinants of health. You can think beyond simply refilling prescriptions or doing physical exams to helping patients to improve their life circumstances as well.

MB: While I'm sure that answer will have some value to many people, it was also very personally motivated, so thanks for the advice. In medical school, we're taught about the various CanMEDS roles: being a professional, being a scholar, being an advocate, and of course, above all else, being a medical expert. When we have sessions regarding advocacy or health systems, some of my colleagues will push back a little and say there are lawyers and social workers for a reason; we have to be physicians. Do you feel as though in order to be a good physician you need to approach your clinical work with a systems or social-determinants perspective? Or is it possible to be a good clinician if you are simply focused on the individual patients in front of you and not at all politically active or interested in the system at large?

RM: There are great varieties in practice. Not everyone is going to be an excellent public advocate, and maybe some of those who are excellent public advocates aren't quite the clinicians that others can be. There are different strengths. However, when you actually look at what we do, it is very difficult to think of any physician not doing, at the very least, the micro level of advocacy: thinking beyond just what they can do in their office, connecting patients to more resources, taking a decent social history, going the extra mile for their patients when it's needed. I like to talk to learners and practising physicians about seeing that as the source of their advocacy, and their clinical knowledge as the source of their strength in advocacy at higher levels, in community and societal levels.

When you are witnessing, for example, refugee patients that aren't able to access medications because of cuts to the Interim Federal Health

Program, it means you fight for that particular patient. But if you're seeing that, you're probably not the only one. So is there a way that you can advocate up the chain so that access is easier to get? Or do you need to be advocating at a national level, the way Doctors for Refugee Care did in response to those cuts? We all see patients, by definition they have vulnerabilities, and we naturally advocate for the individual patient. To take that clinical knowledge and front-line experience and apply it to societal advocacy is very powerful. We should all be keeping that in mind.

MB: So it's great to aim for at least competency in order to be able to serve your patients adequately in each of the roles, but it's difficult for us to expect ourselves to be able to be experts and leaders in absolutely every one of those competencies.

RM: Exactly. I might not be doing original clinical research, but I'm paying attention to the research that's coming out and adjusting my practice accordingly. Maybe I'm being more directly involved in the advocacy level while someone else is keeping an eye out, sharing a Facebook post, giving some money to an organization, because that's what they have time for, that's their level of advocacy. It's appropriate that different people work at different levels. To say that advocacy is not part of what a physician does is to miss a huge opportunity, because we are witnesses to gaps in the system: to patient and community needs and to inequalities. When our advocacy is informed by our current clinical understanding, it is much more powerful.

MB: My advocacy activities actually intensified a little bit when I got into clerkship and started seeing patients on a daily basis. A lot of it had to do with the fact that I had direct motivation. As a pre-clerkship student, when we were primarily in the classroom, I valued advocacy

164

in a theoretical sense, but it wasn't until I was seeing patients day-in and day-out who were unable to afford medications or returning to the emergency department with preventable issues that I fully understood the value of the work and made sure to carve out at least some time for it despite being a medical learner and having all these different responsibilities. Advocacy helps us as much as it can help our patients.

RM: That's a great observation. We teach about the social determinants of health and social accountability in classrooms, but really it's the relationship with patients that is going to drive meaningful advocacy or meaningful work that is directed toward the greatest needs. That's why here in Saskatchewan we started SWITCH, the student-run clinic that works in the inner city, offering after-hours services. Students from medicine, pharmacy, nutrition, dentistry, all the health sciences, and even students from education sometimes are coming down and working. It takes those concepts that are vague – the soft and easy questions on the exam – and makes it clear they are the most important things in the lives of the real people they are meeting. We get students from first year on coming down and getting to know people's stories and know their names and faces. A lot of them become committed to working long term with underserved populations because it means something to them personally.

MB: Do you have any stories that, for you, illustrated the impact of the social determinants of health?

RM: I mentioned that I wrote a book, *A Healthy Society*, that came out in 2012. That was the main idea of that book, taking patient stories and using them to demonstrate how the determinants play out in the lives of individuals. That novel-style approach was much more accessible to people, and it sunk in. If we want to change the frames of how people think about politics and think about social investment, we need to bring it down to that emotional, personal level.

I see patients every day who exemplify the impact of the social determinants of health.

I can think of a patient from this afternoon who is dealing with chronic anxiety. That anxiety is rooted in having been in an abusive relationship, getting mistreated, and being constantly nervous about further mistreatment after having had her self-esteem really knocked down. Before that, she grew up in poverty in a family with tons of kids and family members involved in substance abuse. She's also First Nations and has been part of a population that's been marginalized and has had to deal with the effects of colonization and residential schools. What she presented to me this afternoon were psychosomatic symptoms of anxiety, but really, those are the symptoms of many years of living in poverty, struggling with food security, struggling with family troubles, and those are the result of decades and centuries of marginalization and structural violence that lead to illness at the level of the individual.

■■ **MB:** How do you avoid feeling overwhelmed when you see patients in your clinic who have such complex histories, where so much of what makes them healthy is beyond their control?

■■ **RM:** Some days you just feel overwhelmed, and that's okay. Some days are too big to handle and take a long time to process. I mentioned earlier the balance between front line and big picture. To be able to push for that patient to get the counselling they need, that matters to me. It's important to be able to be part of making things a little bit better for somebody who has struggled a lot. It also means that my involvement in trying to change how we think about politics and trying to decrease the number of people living in poverty, trying to increase access to education or decent housing is grounded in trying to help that one patient, or to help make sure that there are fewer patients in her circumstances in the future. Being able to move back and forth between the individual and the societal is one of the ways that I cope with the enormity of the struggles.

MB: It's somewhat daunting, but also somewhat relieving, to hear that even as a practising physician, you still have those periods where you feel overwhelmed. Especially as a new resident, some days I feel overwhelmed simply because I'm lost, quite physically, in the hospital, and other days, overwhelmed because I've met somebody who's so young but has already led such a complicated and challenging life that it's very hard to see how they'll make it through. Other times I think that it balances out, as we're very privileged to see patients who have overcome a lot and who have an amazing amount of resiliency.

RM: When there is a win, when someone actually listens to your advice, or the treatment that you chose to provide worked, or you got them a social support that made a difference, it's really rewarding. That's where the recharge comes from for sure.

MB: I'm already learning to really celebrate the little victories. At SickKids, a huge proportion of our population are very complex patients, many of whom have issues that have been present from birth. The whole idea of coming to medicine and fixing or curing your patient just doesn't apply in a lot of these cases. These kids will be struggling with some of these challenges throughout their lives. But what I have realized is that if we're able to make even a small difference, even if it's just making somebody well enough so that they can attend school a couple of times a week, that can make a huge difference for patients and their families. Celebrating the small victories of the patients is something that I've started using to deal with some of the more overwhelming and daunting cases.

RM: It's refreshing to talk to someone at your level of training as you're facing those challenges and being overwhelmed on occasion. A career in medicine may mean that you're constantly being overwhelmed by slightly harder things. It doesn't go away, but it gets better as you have a longer view and start to have some experience of the ups and downs. It also sounds like you have a good head on your shoulders and a real understanding of not just the clinical but the social drivers of health. And to me, that is the most exciting thing. When I came into medical school, we were probably even more shocked than your class to learn about the social determinants of health. It was a newer concept, and I was one of the weird outliers who was interested in global health and working with underserved populations. Now it's really become the norm where I teach and across the country. We've seen great advances in terms of the social conscience of medical students and the profession. This year the Canadian Medical Association General Council came out in favour of basic income, divesting from fossil fuels, and expressed 92 per cent support for national pharmacare. This is not the Canadian Medical Association that existed when I was a medical student. It seems our profession has grown into and taken on this mantle of a group that should advocate for the best health of citizens and not just for ourselves. That's very encouraging and very hopeful.

■■ Chapter 15 ■■

Embracing Complexity

James Orbinski (Médecins Sans Frontières/Doctors Without Borders,
Dignitas) – Christopher Charles

Dr James Orbinski is a celebrated humanitarian, physician, and global health scholar. He has extensive field experience with Doctors Without Borders/Médicins Sans Frontières (MSF); he was its international president from 1998 to 2001, and accepted the 1999 Nobel Peace Prize on its behalf. He has since built several globally successful non-governmental organizations. He is a professor of medicine, a bestselling author, a very happy partner, and father of three children (and their part-time chickens) in Guelph, Ontario.

Dr Orbinski is someone I have always looked up to, eagerly reading every published work and attending numerous lectures and forums that he presented at, so it was such a delight and honour to meet him in his office, just around the corner from my own home in Waterloo, Ontario.

■■ **Christopher Charles:** It's so nice to be able to meet with you today. To start things off, I'm wondering if you can help me to understand your interest in the social determinants of health. What has drawn you to social medicine?

■■ **James Orbinski:** The single most important element of any kind of intervention, surely any kind of medical intervention, is effectiveness. In order to understand if X works or not or whether proposed intervention Y will work or not, one has to understand the context and the causal pathways that are at play in determining a particular health or disease phenomenon.

What we know from an evidentiary perspective is that roughly 30 per cent of causality is biomedically determined: that is, the genetics, physiology, anatomy, and pathology of a person and a disease. It's important to have a strong foundation in this area, so that we can disrupt and interrupt it in order to stop a state of disease and recreate a state of ease. The other 70 per cent of causality comes from the social determinants of health. This includes where we live, where we work, what we eat, and how we play. These are major drivers of health status and health outcomes. They are also major factors in understanding causality.

In the way that one seeks to intervene or disrupt from a biomedical perspective, the same thing is true in terms of the social determinants of health. It is really important to understand that these are not mutually exclusive concepts; they are deeply interdependent.

CC: It's similar to the nature-versus-nuture discussion: the nature of the disease is the biomedical component, but the social determinants of health can have a big influence on how that disease plays out, how it is nurtured. Is there one aspect of social determinants that is the most important? Is there one area where you can have the most impact if an intervention is provided?

JO: No, and I have always rejected the question. We live in a kind of a postenlightened world. We have a framework that is logical and linear, and we want to reduce everything to a single answer. Our lived experience tells us that that is not an adequate or appropriate lens for seeing or understanding and engaging the world.

Have you read *Hitchhiker's Guide to the Galaxy*? The driving question of that book is: What is the meaning of life? The protagonist goes on a journey through the cosmos and encounters many, many potential answers, and discovers at the end of the journey that the answer is 42. Then the question is: What does that even mean? It all depends on who is posing the question, and what framework was used to derive the answer.

CC: Things are much more complex now – there are more layers, our worlds are bigger, and yet the world is much smaller. Our understanding of the social determinants of health is very much fortified by our patient contact. Have you cared for a patient recently that illuminates that concept?

JO: I cared for a patient in Malawi about four weeks ago who very much embodies both the biophysical and societal determinants of health. I was at many hospitals and clinics run by Dignitas, and at one I saw a fourteen-year-old girl because of severe malnutrition in the background of stunting. This girl was quite small, with distended belly, edematous hands and feet, rosy-coloured hair, impetigo in a number of different places around her body, and skin that was splitting in several places. All of these indicators point toward profound protein-energy malnutrition.

But what else was embodied in this girl? Well, for one, she's a girl. The largest percentage of people in marginalized groups happens to be women. And if you break that down even further, actually it's girls. There are massive increases in morbidity and mortality relative to boys in many, many places in the world, and that is very much a function of gender. It's important to understand that gender is not some value-neutral term – it is a feature that is embedded in the political, cultural, and societal structure that gives certain privilege or value that is of a lesser quantity to a particular gender than it does relative to another gender. And that is a profoundly important societal determinant of health.

It has different manifestations in different parts of the world, and in different cultures. In this particular case, this young girl – because she was a girl – was far less nourished than her two brothers who were with her, and who although younger than she, were visibly fitter. This little girl was in clinic with her mom, and one of the nurses was chiding her – she was saying to the mother, "How could you leave her in this condition for so long? This is terrible. You're not a good mother." The mother was very upset at being accused of neglecting her daughter but proceeded to explain that their family had been starving because of crop damage as a result of the recent floods in Malawi, which are unequivocally and scientifically without question a consequence of climate change. The mother explained that because of flooding, her house was washed away, her fields were washed away, there was no crop, and therefore no food, and so she had to move away in order to find a job in the market selling little bits and pieces of cutlery, china, and other kitchenware. This girl's mother, as a result of climate change, was also engaging in sex work in order to make money to be able to feed her kids. She had no choice but to do this. Were she not to do this, not only would her daughter be in her current condition, but all of her kids would be in that condition, and some might even have died by this point.

And that's just the beginning. Why did this mother have to walk fifteen kilometres to the clinic with her sick, malnourished children in tow? These distances compound the difficulty of going to seek out medical care. Why isn't medical care seeking out those people who need help and assistance? I asked the clinic manager to explain this further, and he said, "Well, there aren't enough resources." Resources is a word that's become disembodied from the social, political, and economic choices that are made and that determine what funding is available. In Malawi, there is a lack of any type of formal governance framework that determines how resources are used or that ensures that accountability mechanisms are in place so that those funds are used for their intended purpose.

In this particular case, he explained that there are not enough resources, and yet the four major donor governments to Malawi have frozen their aid budgets, despite the incredible need that exists. Why have they done that? Well, fairly recently, in mid-June of 2015, the German government paid for an audit of public accounts in Malawi and found that 32 per cent of all public funding is unaccounted for. In plain English, that means is that 32 per cent of the government budget has gone into people's pockets.

Well, that begs the question: What has happened to the money that was disbursed into government programs? The audit didn't even look at that. It just looked at: X number of dollars came in, Y was spent in government offices and bureaus, and so on, and they found a gaping discrepancy. This provoked a crisis in parliament, and it also meant that budgets for the healthcare system, roads, schools, disaster relief, and everything else was frozen. The nearest local hospital's budget had been cut by 88 per cent. With the amount remaining, you can barely keep the doors open, let alone intervene when needed.

These are the social, political, cultural, and economic factors that drive the health status of that little girl, that child. As a physician, to simply take her weight, examine her heart, and check her potassium and sodium levels, and then start her on an intensive feeding program with a nasogastric tube and four daily feeds for eight days, monitoring for congestive heart failure and looking for beriberi, and all of the other standard stuff that we do – for me simply to do that is not good enough. And for me to not do that, that's equally not good enough. So taking a broader perspective is a necessary starting point to both understanding and then engaging in an attempt to shape and reshape the causes and conditions that determine health status.

■■ **CC:** The problem is laden with complexity. What types of things can you do to look upstream and to prevent that problem in the first place?

■■ **JO:** I would first emphasize that upstream and downstream thinking are not mutually exclusive. That's a big mistake that people make, even today. The battle between public health versus clinical medicine continues. But this is an old story; it's yesterday's battle. The idea that you have to choose between working upstream or downstream is a false choice. If you actually want to be effective, and if you want to participate in institutions that are generally effective, then that kind of false choice has to be tabled. Do you teach a man to fish, or do you feed him for a day? Well it's pretty hard to learn how to fish if you are starving, right?

■■ **CC:** I'm interested to hear what drew you to medicine. I knew that I wanted to practise clinical medicine when I was working in Cambodia as a researcher, and I was going around and collecting blood samples and anthropometric data and spending time in rural and remote communities. During this time, I was constantly approached by people asking, "Can you help my son? Can you help my daughter? My grandmother back at the house has this infection; can you take a look at it?" And I felt like my hands were always tied, and I had no ability to help in a meaningful way. I could do the research, but I didn't have the skill set to help at the individual level. What made you decide to go into medicine?

▮▮ JO: It's just so practical. You can participate in something very specific that can relieve suffering and help individuals or communities overcome a very difficult circumstance. It's really that simple. I like concrete things, and as I have gone through my career thus far, I have recognized increasingly the concreteness of the issues that were previously opaque to me. For example, the importance of research and development platforms, and the governance structures that guide those practices. How is a research question chosen? What gets funded and why? Why hasn't this problem been previously addressed?

The "Lucky Iron Fish" that you developed in response to anemia in Cambodia is a good example. Why is it that someone had not come along and done this? What is it that was different and that made this change and that brought it to the success that it now enjoys? Are you confident that the approach that you are taking is going to have the kind of impact that you want, or are you going to leave that to luck, chance, or faith?

If you just want to treat that patient that you saw in Cambodia, if your hands weren't tied by a lack of knowledge, you could just give them something to help. So you go to medical school. Once you're there, you realize it's not that simple. It's not just, "Oh, you have a cough. Here you go, have some cough syrup." Now that you've had some experience and some training, you realize that action is imbued with domains of knowledge, and that action is not just a response to suffering, it's an informed response to suffering.

There are all kinds of clinical evaluations and ways to understand the nature of medicine and disease. You have to ask yourself, is your patient – the grandmother in that Cambodian village who has been coughing and coughing for fifteen years – going to be able to take nine months of treatment for that terrible tuberculosis? Will she have access to nine months of medication? That act of prescribing a treatment is much more complex, and once you've gone to medical school and acquired the necessary knowledge, you've made the first step.

In my case, now I am further along in my career than you are, and I see it with even more complexity and layers of knowledge and am just beginning to understand what influences those particular choices. The further you go, you can become bewildered by those things – you can think, "Oh god, it's too much," and that is a danger. You can't know everything. If you don't work with others, and you don't respect other people's knowledge and their expertise, then it does become bewildering. Physicians tend to retreat into their own area of specialty – "This is what I know, and this is what I don't. Don't confuse me with all of these other things that I don't understand, and I'm going to be the expert." You must engage in partnerships with others, and in respecting those other professions' knowledge, you might be able to design some kind of intervention that you think rationally has a very high probability of success, based on your understanding of this complex environment. Essentially, you try an experiment. If it doesn't work, you go back and try to analyze why it didn't work. Then you engage yet again. That's actually quite a pragmatic thing, and also quite rewarding and self-satisfying. You're involved in something that can actually matter, and can change a set of circumstances.

■■ **CC:** That's an important consideration. You can tick that effectiveness box, but it has to be acceptable from a cost perspective, and from a patient perspective. Are you asking them to take a pill eight times a day at all different hours? Or is it something that is going to work, that people will take on?

■■ JO: Some of the most important decisions to make when choosing a compound to do research on are your design parameters. What do you want this thing to look like when you're done? Does it match the feasibility requirements of the patient? Not just the biomedical – it has to match that – but it also has to match the requirements of the patient, their environment, and the context in which they live. Do you have to refrigerate the medicine? Is it taken once a day? Twice a day? Three times a day? Is it injectable? Intramuscular? Cutaneous? How do you take this thing? What colour is it? Big bottle, little bottle? It matters – all of it.

■■ CC: Do you remember Virchow's nodes or his triad? He said, "Politics is medicine on a larger scale." What do you think are the political changes in Canada that we would need in order to have better healthcare here on our own soil?

■■ JO: Well, I make a big distinction between health and healthcare. What we typically call healthcare is actually disease-care, and we really have a disease-care system. An approach that would fundamentally change our health status would be a health system as opposed to a disease-care system. Of course, we would still need a system that cared for people who got sick, because people do get disease and they would need relief from pain and suffering. Quite apart from that, we could embed the idea of health in practical operational terms into virtually every facet of our public policy. For example, our transit system, energy policies, and food policies could all be redesigned to maximize health, food security, and environmental sustainability.

We know that as of yet we have failed to address the single greatest driver of health: poverty. In Toronto, 29 per cent of children are going to bed hungry every night. That's incredible. This is the wealthiest society in the history of world, and we fail to see that as a priority. How can we talk about health when 29 per cent of our kids are going to bed hungry? Why are they going to bed hungry? Because their parents can't find proper work, and don't have a guaranteed income.

■■ CC: What do you think physicians or physicians-in-training can do to try and alleviate some of those factors?

■■ JO: The first thing to do is to open our minds and escape the logical, deductive, linear pathway. We need to recognize the complexity and causality of what determines health and recognize our place in that. We need to respect other professions more and work with those who have complementary domains of expertise to co-create interventions. Together, we need to experiment with rationally determined strategies that rely on the best available evidence, the best experience, and the best models, and apply them to our contemporary challenges. That doesn't necessarily mean erasing one's capacity and one's presence. We do know things as physicians that other people don't. But we need to use our knowledge and skills and status to bring that to bear in how we collectively approach problems and interventions.

■■ CC: Whom do you admire most? Is there someone that you think we should be reading? Who inspires you?

■■ JO: There are so many people that inspire me. The people that I find genuinely inspiring are those people who aren't afraid to try. That means being willing to fail, but it also means be driven to succeed. I've seen so many situations that have been perpetually dismissed as irresolvable, beyond our reach. But in many, many situations, I've seen people and had the privilege of working with people who are not afraid to try, who walk into every situation with eyes wide open; people who are willing to fail, but who are ultimately driven to succeed. That's who I admire.

One the people I have long learned from, from a distance, is Vaclav Havel. I find him brilliant and artistically wondrous and rationally a genius – just deeply, deeply inspiring. He would definitely be on my "it" list.

CC: What's driving you right now? What's on your desktop? Dignitas obviously is a big part of your life, but what gets you up every day now?

JO: My big area of interest now is looking at health impacts of climate change and intervention systems that will maximize health. I've been working in Malawi with Dignitas, and we are looking to start a new research initiative on the health impacts of climate change. We are looking at extreme weather events like drought and flood. We do so by examining baseline weather patterns, upon which we can superimpose extreme weather events to look more closely at their impact on food security, infectious disease, and their effect on healthcare systems. Do these types of events disrupt healthcare systems? Yes, certainly they do. But what is the impact on individuals and communities? How is the disaster responded to?

We're collecting this data so that we can create an early warning system that is rooted in community and that uses meteorological data together with data on agriculture, food, crop yields, nutritional impacts, and disease incidence. From there, we can implement appropriate public health surveillance systems and then disaster response systems. The model combines these domains and, allowing for appropriate community inputs, we can assess a situation in the first mile surrounding the disaster, or the epicentre of the disaster, and then we can have relevant outputs, such as early warnings to those living further from ground zero.

▆▆ **CC:** Have you heard the idea that relates the crisis in Syria right now, with climate change – as a direct result of climate change you have migration of families into the city, and the political and civil unrest that has ensued is a direct result of that migration.

▆▆ **JO:** Essentially there was a drought in Syria that started in 2009 that was rather protracted. That led to destabilization of the northern region, and there was a massive migration of people to major cities, and then that group essentially became a marginalized and destabilizing force in a previously stable political architecture of Syria. That's not the first time that's happened. We are seeing this with increasing frequency in many parts of the world.

Darfur is a good example. People talk about war crimes, crimes against humanity, slow-motion genocide – all of which is true. And yes, Mr Al Bashir has been indicted at the International Criminal Court, and he should be brought to trial, and if found guilty he ought to be brought to justice. But that's not a full understanding of the causal variables at play. What drives that conflict in Darfur? Why are people moving to their ethnic and religious affiliations as sources of security? Clearly, the single most important factor is the decreasing availability of potable water and arable land, driven by the impacts of climate change. And that is not going to go away.

Even with the best and most robust treaty agreements, we've

already passed certain critical thresholds, and we will live with those consequences, and they're still not fully evident. We need interventions that help us to adapt better to those inevitable changes that have already started and will continue.

▮▮ Chapter 16 ▮▮

Just Care: From Medicine to Politics in Pursuit of Equity

Jane Philpott (Ministry of Health, Government of Canada) –
Bethany Philpott

Over the course of three decades in medicine, Dr Jane Philpott has seen both health and illness in myriad contexts, and reflected upon the factors that shape wellness for both individuals and society. After completing medical school at the University of Western Ontario and a tropical medicine fellowship at Toronto General Hospital, she worked for nine years in Niger, West Africa. Upon her return to Canada, she practised family medicine in Stouffville and Markham, Ontario, where she became the lead physician of the Health for All Family Health Team and chief of the Department of Family Medicine at Markham Stouffville Hospital.

Dr Philpott's experiences in healthcare reaffirmed her interest in the social determinants of health and dedication to advocacy and ensuring equitable healthcare and health for all. She founded a movement, Give a Day to World AIDS, to raise awareness and funds for HIV/AIDS efforts worldwide. She worked as the family medicine lead for the Toronto Addis Ababa Academic Collaboration, working to develop a family medicine training program in Addis Ababa, Ethiopia. She also completed a Master of Public Health with a global health concentration at the Dalla Lana School of Public Health at the University of Toronto.

Ultimately, Dr Philpott's desire to look upstream and influence the delivery of healthcare itself prompted a move into politics. In the 2015 Canadian federal election, she was elected Member of Parliament for

Markham-Stouffville and was subsequently appointed Canada's Minister of Health. As her daughter, I have had the privilege of watching her career unfold first-hand and have undoubtedly been shaped by her thinking and dedication to service. Now as a medical student myself, I have an even greater appreciation for the work that she has done. In January 2016, I had the opportunity to interview her formally on behalf of Upstream Medicine and explore her commitment to ensuring equity within the Canadian healthcare system.

▨ Bethany Philpott: I'd like to begin by asking what drew you to medicine. I myself took a roundabout way into the field, starting out in social sciences and humanities. I was always interested in the way social, cultural, and political contexts shape people's lives, but it was through experiences with individuals that I was able to see how the body and health, physical and otherwise, also influence people's quality of life on a daily basis. I believe that's what drew me to medicine as a career. What was it that inspired you to pursue medical school?

▨ Jane Philpott: I think my parents were one of the big shaping influences for me. I grew up with my dad, who was a Presbyterian minister, and my mom, who was an elementary school teacher. I was influenced by how they saw themselves as servants of the community. One of the main messages of my upbringing was a sense that I had received a lot in life – lots of opportunities, a good education, and a family that cared about me – and that it was incumbent upon me to make sure that I gave back and chose a career of service. And I was very interested in sciences. In fact, at one point I had considered going into engineering because I always thought that engineers could use science to create great things. But then I began to realize that I really enjoyed working closely with people and eventually realized that one of the best opportunities for being able to spend time with people and serve my community was through medicine.

BP: How has that motivation changed over your career?

JP: One of the things that changed, starting in medical school, was a deeper understanding of issues of equity and inequity in health. I am very grateful for the fact that some of my peers were people who had grown up in other parts of the world. I began to look at the issue of health more broadly and developed an interest in learning about health status in other parts of the world. I went to East Africa for four months in my last year of medical school and worked in western Kenya. That was when I first began to really understand how deeply unfair the world is in terms of the quality of health that people enjoy. I began to understand what it really takes for people to be healthy and why certain populations of the world don't enjoy the same kind of health status that Canadians do. Throughout my training, I continued to learn more about what we now call social determinants of health. I came back from that experience in Kenya with an interest in devoting a portion of my medical career to working in a less-resourced setting, and those experiences internationally have really shaped my understanding of health and of how I can use my career to have an impact on people's health.

BP: Tell me about those experiences working in less-resourced settings. What have you learned about barriers to health and how factors such as geography and income and colonization and all the other social determinants of health shape people's lives and health across the world?

JP: I think the lessons that I've learned working internationally are some of the same things you see in Canada, but perhaps on a different scale. We worked in Niger for about nine years. It continues to be one of the poorest countries in the world economically. With that, there is a tremendous lack of access to education, as well as very serious environmental drivers of health in that it is a country that has chronic drought conditions. All of those things together helped me to realize the huge challenges a country like that faces when trying to make sure that people can live long and well.

■■ BP: You mentioned that the things you saw in Niger are to some degree the same as in Canada but on a different scale. How did you see social determinants of health influence the lives of your patients when you practised family medicine in Markham-Stouffville? Is there an individual story that stands out for you?

■■ JP: I think about a family that I cared for here in Canada. There were many members of an extended family that were part of my practice. This family faced huge challenges in living healthy lives, and the drivers for them, once again, were lack of access to education and problems of literacy and language. They were European immigrants who had trouble, for instance, filling out income tax forms. The matriarch of the family has not learned English very well and is not able to read and write and therefore didn't file income taxes for a number of years. As a result, she had difficulty accessing social services in Canada. The family began to have medical problems and for a variety of reasons weren't able to access medication. Both the mother and father of this family ended up having diabetes that wasn't cared for because of their economic circumstances, even though they were both trying to hold down low-paying jobs. So I saw the impact on the lives of the older members of the family in terms of how their diabetes continued to advance because of lack of access to medication and lack of understanding of their illness condition. I also saw the ripple effect generationally in terms of the challenges faced by their children and grandchildren.

There are many examples of people for whom I could see that the combination of poverty, educational barriers, literacy barriers, and disconnection from social supports meant that their medical conditions became very complicated. This really made me realize that I was only touching the surface of helping them when I addressed the conditions that they presented with in my clinic.

BP: How did seeing people in situations like this and realizing the limitations of what you were able to do within the clinical context shape your practice and your advocacy as a physician? Tell me about the role of a physician as advocate.

JP: Well, there are several ways it shaped me. Family doctors and other healthcare providers can do a lot of basic advocacy every single day with their patients. The kinds of advocacy that I began to get involved with had to do with shaping the care-delivery system. Later on in my practice, I had the privilege of being part of a comprehensive Family Health Team in Ontario, and that's a simple example of how we can provide better care by offering more to our patients than a doctor alone can provide. It was really satisfying to be able to make sure that my patients had access to someone who was an expert in nutrition and diet, and to offer opportunities for them to see a social worker who could address their social needs as well as provide counselling to address issues such as trauma in their lives. That was a way that my practice in Canada began to evolve, but I also started to speak out more about health policy and decisions that were made.

BP: How so?

▮▮ JP: Well, a simple recent example is refugee healthcare. I saw a number of refugees in my practice and realized the challenges that they faced if they didn't have access to care. So I began to speak out about cuts to refugee healthcare. Perhaps more significantly, I began to realize that, as I've said repeatedly, it takes more than medicine to make people healthy. Realizing that if, in fact, the things that affected my patients' lives the most were the economy and the environment and health policy, I began to consider whether perhaps I could do even more if I considered a role in developing and changing health policy, which was what lead me eventually to politics.

▮▮ BP: I want to go back to your comment that there are many things that physicians can do in an office visit to advocate for their patients. Sometimes for medical learners and for those early on in their careers, the concept of advocacy seems very daunting and overwhelming. It can be hard to know where to start. Do you have advice for those entering the field as to how they can be advocates and how they can address the social determinants of health for their patients?

▮▮ JP: Advocacy in medicine at its most basic is being a voice for those whose voices aren't loud enough. During almost every single visit with a patient you may see ways in which that patient is having trouble accessing what they need to be able to be healthy. And I feel very strongly that when healthcare providers recognize that the system is being unfair to one of their patients, the provider has a responsibility to intervene. Some of the most satisfying things I ever had the opportunity to do for my patients were some of the simplest things. Often it involved just picking up the phone.

There are so many other ways, too, that we can advocate for our patients. Some of the other simple, obvious things include establishing clinical settings that are open and welcoming and that will ensure that patients are cared for with respect and dignity. I was always very proud of the teams that I worked with in family medicine. For instance, it's something as simple as the way that a physician sets a tone in their clinic from the moment a patient walks in, and to make sure that your staff realizes that every single person deserves to be treated with the utmost respect and deserves to be listened to. Those are some of the simple things that you can do.

■■ **BP:** It sounds like there's a lot that people can do on that individual basis and in a clinical setting. On the other hand, we also have this metaphor of thinking upstream and trying to solve problems at their source. How has looking upstream impacted the way you work and perhaps your move to politics?

■■ **JP:** Governments play a massive role. One of their most important roles is helping to set the conditions for good health for their citizens. I often say now to my political colleagues that social determinants of health are not solely the responsibility of the health minister but of the whole of government because there isn't a single department of government that doesn't somehow have an impact on people's health. Within health in particular, there are so many policy decisions that will shape the kind of care people have.

■■ **BP:** You're now the federal Minister of Health. What do you hope to achieve? What are your goals for this appointment?

■■ **JP:** I have, of course, the goals that are a part of the mandate that's been given to me by the Prime Minister. I think addressing those issues is going to give me a tremendous opportunity to impact the health of Canadians. Many of my responsibilities have to do with the healthcare system specifically. I've been mandated to negotiate a new health accord with provinces and territories that will include things like improving home care and mental healthcare, as well as making sure that prescription drugs are more affordable. Canadians are rightfully proud of a health system that involves publicly funded health insurance and has been founded on principles such as patients having access to healthcare based on need and not based on ability to pay. Having said that, the context of healthcare delivery has changed a great deal over the last fifty years, and the health policy that undergirds it has not been rigorously evaluated and modernized. So a lot of what I will be working on is looking at how we can continue to uphold the basic principles described in the *Canada Health Act* but make sure we do so in a modern context where healthcare is not provided primarily in hospitals and not provided solely by physicians.

BP: So what are those principles that are shaping your work?

JP: One of the most important principles, of course, is access to care. There continue to be challenges in making sure that access is fair and equitable. We live in an environment where healthcare resources will never be unlimited, and the best example of that is human resources for health. So it's important that we make sure that there will be a fair opportunity for Canadians to access the care providers that they need.

BP: Do you see limited resources then as being the biggest barrier to being able to provide healthcare in the way that we wish?

JP: I actually think it's the structural barriers that are the most challenging. I'm a huge advocate for a healthcare system based on primary care. One of my most influential mentors has been Dr Barbara Starfield. I never knew her personally but read her work, and I feel like every single medical student should read and study the works of Barbara Starfield. I feel ashamed of the fact that I didn't discover her research until many years after I graduated from medical school. If more of us understood the principles of a healthcare system based in primary care, we would be better off as a society. One of my hopes is to work with my political colleagues to ensure that our system is much more patient centred and community based, and a healthcare system as opposed to a disease-centred model. We need to promote health and not just treat illness.

▌▌ BP: This may be a little bit too amorphous to answer, but are you able to describe what a healthy society and a healthy Canada would look like for you?

▌▌ JP: Well, speaking of things that I wish medical learners were taught more about, I would make sure the Declaration of Alma-Ata from 1978 is in the curriculum and written on the minds of medical students. This declaration was an aspirational document that described the goal of "Health for All," founded in the concept of primary care. That document provides some clues to what a healthy society looks like, and it is something that I would like to revisit again in the Canadian context.

"Health for All" requires making sure that citizens have access to the most fundamental determinants of health. Some of the major ones would be economic determinants, such as the ability to earn a living wage and the ability to access good education and ideally advanced levels of education in the modern-day context. Those are very important for delivering health, as are social policies that will make sure that people have fair access to opportunities. There is a big, long list of what would be necessary, but those are some of the most important items.

■ BP: What else would you add to the reading list for medical learners? What other things have been influential in shaping your perspective?

■ JP: If I were to go back again, the other area I would talk about would be ethics. I'm not necessarily talking about bioethics or clinical ethics, but more some of the grounding principles. Speaking about the heroes in the system, I would include people like Dr Solomon Benatar from South Africa, whose writing has been very influential in understanding health from a global ethics point of view. In fact, I'd say that the readings that have most shaped my career are not from the health sector, but stories about social justice – books like Nelson Mandela's *Long Walk to Freedom*, or Adam Hochschild's *Bury the Chains*, which describes the end of the slave trade.

■ BP: Are there other current role models you admire?

■ JP: I would mention somebody like Dr Lynn Wilson, who's the former chair of the Department of Family and Community Medicine at the University of Toronto and who has been a tremendous mentor. I look to people like Jeff Turnbull and Chris Simpson of the Canadian Medical Association. Stephen Lewis is not a doctor but has been hugely influential in my career. People that I look up to so much now in the healthcare system include Samir Sinha, Meb Rashid, Gary Bloch, and of course, Danielle Martin.

■ BP: What is it about them? What traits do these people share that you would emulate?

■ JP: I think the most important thing is that these people have an equity lens, and their fundamental driver is making sure that the health system is fair.

BP: So it's about equity and providing health for all?

JP: That's probably the most important thing. Having said that, one of the things I like to emphasize is that injustice anywhere is a threat to justice everywhere. That line is taken from Martin Luther King, Jr., but I often paraphrase in the health context and say that ill health anywhere is a threat to wellness everywhere. What that translates into is that when we're really looking at trying to make sure that the health system is equitable, it benefits everyone if we make sure that the most vulnerable among us have access to great healthcare. A society that cares for its most vulnerable is ultimately a healthy and prosperous society, and the more inequality in the system, the more we'll all suffer. Does that make sense?

BP: It definitely makes sense. The challenge is how you get everyone to see that. So my final question comes back to you and how you are able to take care of yourself. You've accomplished a lot, and you work hard. Where is the room for balance and self-care? How do you maintain that?

JP: A lot of my balance comes from my family. I have an extremely supportive husband. I make sure that I get plenty of time at home with my family. Some of my favourite times of all are when I get to hang around home with my husband and kids. My favourite holidays of all are going to the cottage and spending time with both our immediate family and our extended family. I make sure I get enough sleep and enough downtime to relax and read.

▪▪ Chapter 17 ▪▪

It's Our Duty

Meb Rashid (Doctors for Refugee Care) – Ben Langer

On July 1, 2012, the Government of Canada made major cuts to the Interim Federal Health Program (IFHP), which since 1957 had provided healthcare and extended benefits to all refugees and asylum seekers in Canada. At the time, I was a medical student far from home, in Israel/ Palestine working with Physicians for Human Rights – Israel on their own asylum-seeker project. The first time I saw Dr Meb Rashid was on a YouTube video as he was making a passionate deposition before Parliament on behalf of refugee health. Truly inspired and outraged, it wasn't long before I was home and launching myself headlong into the struggle for refugee health in Canada led by Doctors for Refugee Care, an organization co-founded by Dr Rashid.

I was astonished at the courage of these doctors who used their privilege to speak up for those whose voices were being stifled and whose stories were being erased. That fall, I became the national officer for Human Rights and Peace for the Canadian Federation of Medical Students and had the privilege of partnering with Doctors for Refugee Care throughout a year of refugee health advocacy. Dr Rashid, an excellent clinician who directs the Crossroads Refugee Clinic at Women's College Hospital in Toronto, was then and still remains at the centre of the movement. Always calm, collected, and diligent about the facts, Dr Rashid is a real inspiration to me and a role model of how I want to do my medical and advocacy work. We were able to connect late one work night over the phone.

■■ Ben Langer: The two concepts that form the focus of this book are thinking and acting upstream and the social determinants of health, and I wanted to know whether you think in these terms when you think of your work.

■■ Meb Rashid: Everyone I see now is a recently arrived refugee, and we're often seeing them within days of arrival, so obviously, immigration status is important, but many people arrive with absolutely nothing. Other issues like housing, access to resources, food security, all of these issues really undercut people's health status on arrival. A lot of the people we are seeing are housed in refugee shelters, but fortunately their trajectory is such that they're getting their immigration status resolved quite quickly. Thus, a social determinants of health approach is a really significant part of the work that we're doing.

■■ BL: Tell me a little bit about how you came to be where you are, what the moments were that shaped your own journey, and who the people were who influenced you along the way.

■■ MR: I graduated quite a long time ago, and spent about seven years as a locum here in Toronto. I did some work in Nicaragua, Zimbabwe, and Tanzania. After seven years as a locum, I had an opportunity to take over someone's practice at a community health centre focused on immigrants and refugees. It was a time in my life where I'd just had a kid, so I decided to take the job. When I started there, probably 75 per cent of the practice was people who were undocumented. Over the course of the seven years I was there, that changed, and about 95 per cent of our new patients were newly arrived refugees. It had become clear to me through my time at the community health centre that there was a tremendous interest among medical students and residents to learn more about refugee health, and there was also a tremendous paucity of literature guiding clinicians working in the refugee health sector in Canada. When I left the community health centre at the end of 2009, I'd seen refugee clinics sprout up all across the country, but there wasn't yet a clinic in Toronto devoted exclusively to the needs of refugees. I approached a few academic sites and Women's College was one that was eager to push forward with a refugee health clinic. Five years ago, we opened up Crossroads Clinic at Women's College Hospital, and that's where I've been since.

As to what got me interested in the work, you know I've always been fascinated by some of the medical issues that confront newly arrived immigrants. I have a bizarre interest in certain parasites and malaria and tuberculosis and things of that sort that I'd seen more of overseas. But I think more compelling was really people's stories. You would see people who had lived through quite unimaginable trauma and had demonstrated such amazing resiliency. Having arrived in Canada, the majority of people I see have a tremendous desire to put their lives back together and contribute to society. I got completely drawn to working with that population.

As far as people who influenced me, there are some amazing people working in the community health centre [CHC] sector here in Toronto. People like Kevin Pottie, who started in the CHC sector and now he's in Ottawa. There's another physician named Jim Sugiyama who you might not have heard of, a very soft-spoken man here in Toronto and just an amazingly devoted physician. There are some really wonderful people doing some really interesting work, and I had the opportunity to be mentored by some of them, particularly in my first ten years of practice. In refugee health, there are fantastic people all throughout the country; it's a wonderful community to work with. Philip Berger is someone else who I've really come to know well over the past four or five years. He has cunning political instincts; I've certainly learned a tremendous amount from him.

More than anything, it's the patients who really drive my work. I always say that I have the best job in the city. There isn't a day goes by that I don't run into somebody who has lived through something that if you put it on the screen no one would believe it. And they continue to forge forward with their lives, and it's an amazing thing to share with them.

▮▮ BL: When I first started seeing newly arrived patients, refugees and others, there were a few whose stories, personalities, and resolve just stuck in my mind. I was wondering if there are any individual stories you have that you could share, which highlight the challenges for newcomers and refugees in coming to a place like Canada and forging a new life.

▮▮ MR: There are literally hundreds. I remember a woman I met years ago who arrived pregnant, with her husband. She was a journalist in her home country. She was left for dead twice – buried up to her neck in sand, once by one side of a conflict, and the other time by the other side – was found on both occasions, and navigated her way to Canada with her family on a tortuous route. She was still dealing with those scars through her pregnancy. I got to know her well over the next three or four years as she slowly put her life together, but then I left the practice. Two or three years ago, I got a call from her – she invited me to a ceremony she was having to celebrate her anniversary. She'd gone back to school and graduated and was working, and her little one was now three or four years old. This is so typical of so many of the stories we hear of people who go through horrible trauma – you know it wasn't easy for her when she arrived. She came as a government-sponsored refugee so her immigration status wasn't an issue, but she really struggled in the transition. But if you give people enough time and supports, they demonstrate resiliency. She's happy here, she's thriving, she has a family that she adores, and there are so many stories like that.

BL: Knowing someone who has gone through that journey, you really get a sense of how important it is to have supports in place. In that vein, I want to talk about the time when we first met, which was in the wake of the 2012 changes in the IFHP and the passing of Bill C-31 [which restricted refugee rights to appeal decisions made by the minister of immigration on whether their home countries were safe and allowed for their summary deportation] here in Canada. At that time, I had learned a little about refugee health, and I knew that there were special challenges that they faced, but I thought that Canada was an open-door country that had a policy, and a legacy, of caring for refugees. This was the first time I was exposed to the real politics of immigration and refugees, and it was a bit shocking. How have the politics of refugee health changed over the course of your career, and what we can learn from those changes?

MR: I've been working with refugee populations since I graduated and really in depth for the last ten to twelve years. Until about 2009 or 2010, I hadn't seen dramatic changes in government policies toward refugees. There was some fine-tuning. For example, I was involved in the advisory committee for the IFHP in 2008 and 2009. I remember sitting with some clinicians, but also a number of people from Citizenship and Immigration Canada, and being incredibly impressed by their desire to make the program work, to make it more efficient. They really spoke like advocates. There was a tremendous group of people really trying to do their best to ensure

197

that people did adjust well here in Canada.

That has changed in the last four to five years. The rhetoric around refugee migration has changed completely; the focus is on portraying refugees as cheats, as people who are ripping off the system. In terms of health insurance, the IFHP has been in place since 1957, and it had provided comprehensive care for decades. To see that cut was just unnecessary and excessively cruel. The Federal Court has stated quite clearly that the cuts disadvantaged people who everyone agrees are already severely disadvantaged. The Federal Court decision also spoke very clearly about the rhetoric that had been used by the former Conservative government. There had certainly been an emphasis on changing the refugee processing system and changing refugee health in the last five years. A lot of those changes were incredibly regressive.

BL: My other experience of refugee health was in Israel, where over the last ten years about 60,000 people have come to Israel, mostly on foot or with human traffickers through Sinai, mostly from Eritrea and Sudan. They have suffered greatly on the journey, but then also when they arrive in Israel they are essentially labelled infiltrators and don't receive any sort of status or healthcare. Around the world, there is a shift in rhetoric, and it really seems that what is happening in Canada is part of a global shift in the discourse around refugees and migration. I was wondering if you had contact with other people in other countries, and if there was anything of a strategy of countering that changing narrative at a more global level.

MR: I am in contact with physicians from Spain and Australia and elsewhere, and we all agree that there has been this push to the bottom, but through that there are also examples of countries that have been incredibly generous. Sweden has accepted a staggering number of asylum seekers in the last few years. That's not to say that there haven't been issues, there haven't been conflicts, or internal angst. Germany also, they're anticipating over 100,000 in 2015. So there have been examples of countries that have been models for accepting refugees and acknowledging the contributions refugees can make to their societies as well.

But I agree, the tone has certainly changed, and these are not times where generosity toward refugees or migrants is commonplace. This is going to be one of the great challenges of our generation. There are particularly dark times right now with the number of Syrian refugees in particular. There is such inequity in the world that more and more we're seeing people who have had to endure horrors, endure famine, endure economic atrocities, and who recognize that there are places in the world where people can live comfortably. The disparities are becoming more striking: more and more people are able to move, or at least are aware of this dichotomy, and we're seeing this everywhere. We're hearing again about building a wall between Mexico and the United States, or hearing about Fortress Europe, but as long as you have this inequity, people are going to come, there's no way around that. So it's a tremendous challenge for our generation, and I don't think there are any easy answers; certainly building walls is not going to be the answer. I do notice that there is a global trend of making it more difficult for refugees and refugee claimants, and there are many people struggling against it, but you know in the end, I haven't heard of a concerted movement that's been effective in leveraging opposition to those trends.

▮▮ **BL:** The vast majority of refugees never make it to a country like Sweden or Canada or Germany; they're displaced in another country nearby. For instance, the number of Somalis in Kenya, the number of

Iraqis and Syrians in Jordan is in the millions. What sort of action can we take to address the major challenge of internally displaced persons and people who are seeking refuge in countries where they just don't have the capacity to resettle the number of people who have arrived?

MR: Close to 90 per cent of refugees end up in the developing world, in countries like Tanzania and many other countries that just don't have the infrastructure. Despite everything you hear about places like Europe and North America being overrun by refugees, the true burden is on countries like Pakistan, Jordan, and Lebanon. It's hard to deny that these countries really struggle with developing the infrastructure for accommodating such large migrations in such a short period of time. It's hard to get around the issue of resources. You need to be able to put water together, develop communities, find a way for people to develop small economies, and more and more you hear of organizations struggling to keep up. It's almost obscene to hear the kinds of things you hear from Canada when there are millions of Afghans in Pakistan, millions of Iraqis in Jordan.

BL: Medicine can be a very demanding career all on its own, and family medicine especially has a wide and ever-expanding knowledge base. How do you balance advocacy work with medical practice, and what advice would you give to someone eager to be both an excellent advocate and an excellent physician?

MR: It really has to go hand in hand. If you're going to advocate, you have to be a good clinician, because it's quite easy to tear people apart if they're not practising good medicine. If you're sticking your neck out for a particular issue, you want to make sure that your medicine is sound.

Also, if you're working with high-needs populations, it's really impossible not to advocate for them. Different people do it in different ways. For some people, it might be helping people find housing or dealing with a problematic landlord; for others, it's pushing policy changes on certain issues. My experience has been that it certainly helps to have allies, making sure that you develop coalitions. But, I've never felt any resistance from colleagues, not once. I was at Women's College Hospital six months when I had to call my chief and say, "Tomorrow I'm going to go occupy some government buildings." But it's never been a problem.

What I think all of us struggle with is time. There are a lot of different pulls, and being able to balance all of that becomes a struggle. But it's really hard to do family practice and not advocate for your patients. There's no easy answer, but it is possible, and I'd even go so far as to say that it's part of our duty.

■■ **BL:** Often people involved in advocacy have a hard time giving themselves a break, especially when they see that the people they're advocating for aren't allowed that sort of break for self-care. So how do you navigate that emotional landscape and take care of yourself?

■■ **MR:** I'm in a fortunate position in some ways because a lot of the people I see have fled from their horrors. For every horrific story you hear, and you certainly hear them, there's also so much optimism. There's a tremendous desire for people to put their lives back together. I see so much resilience in the people I deal with, despite the hardships they have suffered, and I've always found it more inspiring than destroying. It also makes a really big difference to have a community you can share your stories with. I've got great networks of people who share similar interests, who are interested in hearing these stories. I've also got a partner who is drawn to a similar type of work. That really helps, so you're not carrying that weight yourself. It makes a huge difference, to be able to share a little of that hardship.

■■ BL: What do you think is next for refugee health in Canada? What are the areas we need to work on, and how can we get there?

■■ MR: One is detention, and I think there has been some attention drawn to this by the United Nations High Commissioner for Refugees. Certainly, there really is no reason why somebody should be forced into detention upon arrival or even at the endpoint of their trajectory in the refugee system. Another issue that's come up, and it's a more difficult one, is family reunification. We're seeing a number of people who have been accepted, but their families are still living through horrendous things, and it's sometimes taking two or three years to get them here. We've known people who have died in that time, and we've known children who've been sexually abused while awaiting this process. A third issue is, of course, just plain numbers.

■■ BL: I think it's time for my cohort, my generation, to step in and step up, and see where we can play a role. Do you have any last advice for a resident or medical student who is looking to get involved and is looking to be a good advocate?

■■ MR: Philip Berger always says you have to be tremendously diligent about the facts. You've got to know the issue cold, and you can't exaggerate. You've got to be true to what's going on. The other thing I've learned from Philip is to be completely unrelenting. Find something you feel passionate about and learn everything about it, then really stay true to the facts.

◼◼ Chapter 18 ◼◼

Spaces to Live, Work, and Play

Michael Schwandt (Public Health Activist) – Natasha Goumeniouk

Dr Michael Schwandt trained in the public health and preventative medicine residency program at the University of Toronto, and within that did family medicine training and then the public health part. He is currently Deputy Medical Health Officer at Saskatoon Health Region, and also does teaching and research at the University of Saskatchewan.

◼◼ **Natasha Goumeniouk:** Can you tell me a bit about what you do?

◼◼ **Michael Schwandt:** The programs that I run are giving public health and medical advice direction to the environmental public health programs. That involves everything from the reactive side of public health practice that could be responding to, say, an outbreak or a cluster of illness that might be related to environment, say a food-borne outbreak, to the more strategic long-term aspect, which is trying to plan for healthy environments, looking at what we can do to make cities healthier, the health effects of climate change, and other such issues.

◼◼ **NG:** And the courses you're involved in and your research is geared toward that as well?

◼◼ **MS:** Yes, the research is exactly that, trying to understand how health equity can play out in some of those areas. One area that we're involved in here is injury prevention in Saskatoon, looking at health urban planning to limit injuries and death for pedestrians, cyclists, and

203

motorists as well. We see that the rates of injury are higher for certain areas of the city than others, and this often follows socio-economic status. We're really trying to understand those different gradients of health for different determinants, and then act on that. We're learning to see health inequities and what we can do about it.

■■ **NG:** Our medical class just got the opportunity to do simulation of living with less in Kingston. It was quite an interesting challenge. The different rooms in our medical building were turned into Ontario Works [a provincial support program] housing offices, healthcare clinics, and everyone was given a different character whose problems we had to embody. Then, throughout the exercise, we actually met the so-called character, the person whose life story we had been enacting.

Overall, it was met positively, and although some students felt we were trivializing the issue of poverty, I think it was a good way for students to learn hands-on what resources are available and what they could do with them. Of course, conditions in Kingston aren't necessarily going to be the same as in Saskatoon or in other parts of Canada. What do you think are the most important forces shaping the lives of those in your community?

■■ **MS:** I would certainly say that poverty is one of the biggest causes of ill health, and it's something that can make other causes of illness worse. We see so many impacts of poverty, as you would have seen during the exercise you described, at the point of access to health services. Transportation, access to child care, employment, all of these things impact access to health services, but also affect the more upstream process of health, including our material ability to access healthy foods, housing, medications, opportunities for physical activity.

I've been interested in what our environment allows for as well. If you look at the community I'm sitting in right now in downtown Saskatoon, it's been the subject of a lot of studies about food security and has been described as a food desert, as there isn't necessarily access to food at any cost in the nearby vicinity. This gets into what the cities that we live in look like, how are they planned, and how they facilitate good health. Looking at environmental health is increasingly intertwining with health-equity issues, and we're finding that a lot of these issues of poverty can really dovetail with the surrounding environment. Whether that's access to healthy food, the presence of contaminants, healthy air, healthy land, all of these things seem to interact quite a lot.

Thinking of this issue of healthy cities, one thing that can really impact people's health is transportation. Active transportation or the presence of useful public transportation – a lot of cities where there's not good access to those things, that's going to impact on access to healthy foods and employment. If someone isn't able to get to employment or juggle that along with say, child care, access to medical services, or education, that can be a huge detriment to health.

■■ **NG:** Can you tell me more about your personal experiences with the members of the community who are facing health challenges?

■■ **MS:** One issue that is more day-to-day is doing the public-health inspections of housing. Right now it's safe to say that there is a shortage of safe and affordable housing in the city, so often we are called to inspect the public health conditions of some of the housing. Unfortunately, a lot of the time it's a really negative picture, with what could be an outright risk for injury in the short term, and long-term elevated risks for infectious disease, and the mental health and social effects of living in substandard housing, especially for children. These conditions have a downstream effect on people's ability to afford to engage in employment or education or training. Somebody who doesn't have a safe, healthy place where they can spend time, it's not a healthy place to develop as a child.

Housing as a determinant of health is something we see all the time. We try to work with landlords to bring housing up to par, while doing more long-term advocacy for an actual strategy toward housing, whether that's at a level of cities or provinces or even a national housing strategy.

That's extremely important, and when you're looking at someone's ability to access primary care, specialist care, any aspect of the health system, it's absolutely essential to have a house or home to begin with. We take this "Housing First" approach. In cases when treating mental health or addiction, you're not going to succeed without ensuring that that person has a home, so one of the first things you have to do is work with different partners to get someone in a good housing situation.

▌▌ **NG:** So that "Housing First" approach sounds very similar to a "Health in All Policies" idea, where you want that to play into every aspect of policy decision-making, because that's where health really starts. In a general sense, what do you consider a good political culture that produces health outcomes?

▌▌ **MS:** I think that having health or health-determining conditions as one of our bottom lines for all policy decisions is key. The same way we look at the median economic impact (and for the media, that's often the main posted outcome of a policy decision), looking at the health outcome can be among the key considerations. Whether that's a city-level consideration about transport or urban planning, or a provincial decision about social services or income support, or a federal decision that could affect our health system, for all of these things, we need to make sure that people's health and well-being are right up there in terms of the outcomes we look at, so that we're not just adding up the dollars and cents.

In addition to that, although the cost-benefits aren't always talked about in the media, having this "Health in All Policies" approach is financially prudent. In the long run, there are actually cost savings. For example, in a city with a good active-transport plan, it's not just about saving money for the people who walk and cycle and have those immediate benefits, it actually saves the health system a great deal of money in terms of chronic disease and injuries. Putting health into those considerations will show us where some of those payoffs can be.

NG: I'm from Vancouver originally, and these past couple of summers we've had a lot of debate in the city over bike lanes being put in and commuter bridges losing car lanes to pedestrians and cyclists. This initially met a lot of resistance, but I'm hoping that it works out long term for the city in that more people are encouraged to bike and walk to work despite the rainy weather.

MS: Vancouver has made a lot of big steps. Also, this will hopefully move people into types of transport that aren't carbon emitting, which has implications for climate change in the longer run as well. There are lots of different benefits to taking that kind of approach.

NG: Do you have anything in particular that drew you into public health? What made you decide to take that path at the University of Toronto, and what brought you to where you are now?

MS: Like many medical students, I liked it all when I was going through school, and the best of family medicine or emergency medicine were really inviting to me. But I found myself increasingly looking at what were the causes of the medical condition I was looking at, and always wanting to take one step back or one step upstream in terms of prevention. I think that's what led me to public health, trying to look at entire communities. Being able to work with patients directly but also considering a bigger picture and getting to look at those things in a broader, societal way was an important piece. That's the cornerstone of what the public health field is all about.

NG: During your medical education, did you feel like you were supported in your learning? When you wanted to take a step back, was this encouraged?

MS: Oh yes! A lot of medical education and training deals with downstream outcomes, which are also absolutely critical. You need curative medicine, and a lot of important preventative medicine happens in those contexts as well. Increasingly, medical schools are recognizing both the immediate aspects and the larger social-determinants role in the curriculum. When I was a medical student, they talked about it less than they do now, and that's certainly increased over recent decades. I found some really great mentors in my own training, and with successive generations it only becomes a bigger part of training and practice.

NG: Do you have any suggestions for how best to educate student learners about the role we play and how we can impact the system upstream?

MS: I think that with all of us, medical trainees and practitioners, it's an action-oriented field, and we want to be able to see that we are helping the patient in an immediate way. Making those connections and seeing an immediate impact can be very helpful. A lot of our experience with clinical doctors and the training we do in medical school is seeing what you can do today to adjust the determinants of health for a given patient, like a direct referral to another service or an agency, but also linking that to what could make that picture better for other patients in a similar situation. So often we think that these are big systems and we don't have a role in them, but for a variety of reasons, physicians do have a significant voice at the table and have a special understanding that comes from direct contact with many patients. We have some opportunity or even responsibility to take these lessons to the bigger picture, because we have that knowledge and a pretty significant voice in society.

NG: I'm someone who gets very personally involved with the cases I see. Do you find that's the case for you, too? When you're dealing with all these upstream issues, do you ever feel overwhelmed or exhausted by what you're encountering?

MS: Oh, certainly. One of my formative experiences in med school was when a patient got admitted to internal medicine for quite a long while. He was discharged to the community, but it was clear that his housing situation was unstable at best, and it was a reasonable understanding by the team that this patient would not be able to manage his co-morbidities in the situation that he was being discharged to. There I was, a medical student on the team, feeling that we should address this. This is something that really directed me toward public health, trying to create systems where the patients and physicians don't experience this helplessness. Just as we have clinical pathways to make sure that patients get the right tests and the right treatment, we need pathways to make sure that these other determinants are addressed so that it can help to deal with some of these feelings. Often we realize that our training is just a small part of the many things that are influencing health. So you can have that feeling of being a small piece, but by really making yourself aware of the teams and the systems around, you can address that kind of feeling.

NG: So you're suggesting looking at these social determinants as a factor just like anything else, rather than separating it out and creating its own category. It's a base criterion we need to look at.

MS: Exactly. If someone has a fractured hip or a complication of diabetes, we wouldn't consider our management complete until we fully addressed the surgical or pharmacological aspects, and the social aspects may be just as much a part of our care because they can certainly be just as influential in terms of outcomes.

Chapter 19

Bringing Upstream to the Mainstream

Chris Simpson (Canadian Medical Association) – Jonathon Herriot

Dr Chris Simpson is past-president of the Canadian Medical Association (CMA) and chief of cardiology at Kingston General Hospital/Hotel Dieu Hospital and Queen's University. During his term, he continued the leadership of previous CMA presidents in emphasizing the importance of the social determinants of health and including this in his advocacy efforts. As the voice of Canadian physicians to the federal government, his focus on the social determinants of health can leverage a broad spectrum of policy changes that can make a real difference to the lives of Canadians. The CMA's involvement in this work represents an exciting shift in Canada toward upstream medicine becoming mainstream medicine.

Through my four years of medical school at the University of Saskatchewan, I have became fascinated with the impact of social circumstance on the health and happiness of Canadians. This has led to a keen interest in how physicians and policy-makers can break down social barriers to good health. I first crossed paths with Dr Simpson when I invited him to speak at our annual University of Saskatchewan Health Innovation and Public Policy Conference in 2014. He spoke to hundreds of students and faculty about the seniors' care crisis in Canada and the importance of advocacy in medicine. In September of 2015, I spoke with Dr Simpson to discuss the importance of the social determinants of health in his clinical and leadership work, and the need for federal leadership to move beyond the status quo of health policy in Canada.

▮▮ Jon Herriot: It's obvious in your advocacy work with the Canadian Medical Association that you have an interest in the social determinants of health. Could you tell us a bit about what draws you into the area?

▮▮ Chris Simpson: Well, the CMA was on a path to focusing on the social determinants of health even before I arrived on the scene, and it was during Anna Reid's presidency that it really received top billing. It was the meeting in Yellowknife where Sir Michael Marmot came over, and it really ignited the leadership around the role that doctors can play in addressing the social determinants of health. I think we've been relatively successful raising the profile of the social determinants of health. Any time an organized medical group, which is necessarily going to be slow to change, embraces a progressive cause like the social determinants of health, that really raises the profile in the mainstream and helps to facilitate change. So my interest was really piqued by the fact that the organization was interested in it.

▮▮ JH: Since I entered medical school in 2012, I have seen a more progressive face of the CMA. The report on the social determinants of health town halls, "What Makes Us Sick," was quite exciting. Now that the CMA is talking about the social determinants of health, what do you see as their role in getting a "Health in All Policies" approach to be adopted in Canada?

▮▮ CS: The social determinants of health inform all of our policy-making, particularly around advocacy. When we appear at parliamentary committee meetings and senate committees, our work on advocacy on social determinants of health is always there, it is always specifically mentioned, and it is always in our recommendations. This is not one of these things that was a CMA project for a year and then forgotten about. It has fundamentally changed the organization, and I expect that it will always critically inform our work. The other thing that is really interesting is the role that the CMA has been able to take internationally on the social determinants of health. The best example of that was the conference that we co-hosted with the British Medical Association several months ago where Sir Michael Marmot – who is arguably the intellectual and emotional leader of the cause worldwide – really lauded the CMA for being "best in class" in terms of medical organizations. He was able to cite several projects by Canadian physicians that were being highlighted by the CMA, projects like the work that Ryan Meili does and the work that Gary Bloch does at St. Mike's in Toronto and so on.

JH: Do you predict that with different leadership it could ever swing the other way, or do you think that the CMA has become more progressive and more interested in the social side of medicine forever?

CS: I think it's a permanent change. I know in the past, when certain presidents have been at the helm of CMA, there has been a perception – sometimes a reality as well – that things swing in a slightly different direction. But the organization now is far more strategic, and the progressive nature of the organization is permanently embedded.

JH: Good to hear. You mentioned Sir Michael Marmot. Is there anyone else that you would say is a role model or someone who has inspired your approach to leadership and advocacy work with the CMA?

CS: I'm inspired by a lot of Canadians. There are people like Monika Dutt in Cape Breton, Ritika Goel and Gary Bloch in Toronto, and of course Ryan Meili, whom I was so impressed with that I brought him to Kingston to do a medical grand rounds. I find him just such a compelling, sincere, and authentic guy on these issues. There are many more doing great work, but in terms of walking the talk, those four are really great examples of social leadership in medicine in Canada.

▇▇ **JH:** I couldn't agree more. I was able to work with Dr Bloch and Dr Goel while I was in Toronto in the last couple of weeks. Those physicians you listed, they are very excited about the social determinants of health, trying to do research around it, and to find their role in improving the social determinants of health. Do you have any ideas about how we could get that to spread to all family physicians or all physicians across the country?

▇▇ **CS:** The key is some of the practical things they are doing. If you look at the poverty assessment tool used by people like Ritika Goel and Danyaal Raza that was adopted by the Ontario College of Family Physicians, these are practical bedside tools that allow the average physician to move beyond a social conscience toward actual activism. It allows them to do something in their practice to help recognize the social gradient of disease and to do something about it.

When Gary Bloch talks about prescribing money, it is a headline grabber, and everybody says, "What?" Then when they actually hear what he is talking about, they say, "You know, that actually makes sense. You treat poverty like a disease. That is a paradigm that I am familiar with. I can do that." We always talk about basic science being translated to clinical work, but this is more like social science being translated into traditional medical-speak. It makes it familiar and comfortable for physicians who were trained classically to get into that space.

▇▇ **JH:** You've been doing a great deal of advocacy around seniors' care. On the surface, seniors' care doesn't seem like a particularly upstream issue. Can you tell me why you think this is an upstream issue?

CS: It is very much an upstream issue because it definitely does bring in many aspects from the social determinants of health discussion, including things like the percentage of seniors who are living below the poverty line being at the highest rate in Canada that it has been in almost forty years. When you have seniors who have to choose between paying for drugs and paying their rent, then it becomes a very important issue. Things like poverty, housing, nutrition, access to healthy foods – all of these are at least as important to seniors as they are to others. It becomes very important to think about those upstream factors in the context of a seniors' strategy. This has been the greatest barrier to getting everybody on board with a seniors' strategy, because they think all we are talking about is hospitals and doctors and healthcare. But if we are talking about helping seniors age well, then we very quickly bring in all those upstream issues, and we realize that to deliver the best quality of care at the best value for taxpayer dollars, investing in those social determinants is money very well spent.

JH: Besides seniors' care, what other policy ideas aren't being talked about enough in the mainstream election cycle that would lead to greater health in Canada?

CS: It is not nearly as glamorous to say this, but we need a better structure for having these conversations. Right now, we have ten provinces and three territories, all of which I have to believe have leaders whose hearts are in the right place but have different solutions for slightly different problems. We are far less than the sum of our parts when everybody is working differently and not learning from each other or figuring out how to come together to scale things up.

That is why we believe that the federal government needs to be at the health table, because they are the only ones that can play this unifying role and set national standards, or at the very least present an aspirational goal. For example, if we want to say in five years that we will have the best wait-times in the industrialized world – right now we have among the worst – that can only be done with a national recognition of the problem and national development of a solution. Or if we said we want to be the country that has the fewest number of preventable hospital complications, these things can only be accomplished with a unified voice.

You can identify any number of upstream or downstream things that need to be fixed, but it cannot be done with strict ideological adherence to this federated model using the constitution as an excuse. Siloism is not the way to fix this stuff, and it is far too Balkanized. Whenever we talk about any issue, we always try to bring it back to "this is the problem, this is what needs to be fixed," but what are the structures and the organizational levers that we have to make it happen? This federal-provincial divide always seems to be the barrier. David Naylor's report talked about putting this kind of governance infrastructure in place so that we can address these problems more effectively than we have been doing so far.

We can all say that we want a national pharmacare plan – it's pretty hard to find a Canadian that doesn't agree with that – but how can you do that with a federal government that's not at the table? It's virtually impossible. We have seen the Council of the Federation make attempts to come together, but they can only pick off the low-hanging fruit, like drug prices. There needs to be a common, unifying force that helps to set those goals and establish accountability in solving them.

■■ **JH:** You're a cardiologist in Kingston, Ontario. Why do the social determinants of health matter to your practice even in your acute care hospital setting?

■■ CS: I see patients all the time that, without poverty-reduction screening tools and knowing what to ask, would fly under the radar. I have learned a lot from others about how simple questions can really unmask a lot of really important issues. The scenario I see most commonly is in people who, after heart attacks, are recommended to take a cocktail of medications that includes Aspirin, Plavix [a blood thinner], a beta blocker [an anti-hypertensive], ACE inhibitors [another anti-hypertensive], and a statin [a cholesterol-lowering medication]. This is the evidence-based regimen for reducing mortality and improving quality of life after a heart attack. But when you add up the costs of those, if it's not covered under the drug plan or the Ontario Drug Benefit, then the cost can be $250 to $300 a month. There are a lot of people who simply cannot afford that. You can refer them to a social worker, who can sometimes help, sometimes cannot, but I sometimes find myself actually having the conversation saying, "If you can only afford $150 a month, these are the medications I would stop taking first." I actually tell them, "It's better to take four out of five than none at all, and if you have to drop one, this is the one that is probably going to have the least positive impact." It sounds ridiculous that a physician would have to say that, but I have to believe that I am doing good when I recognize the reality of the impact that their social circumstance imposes on them. The solution, of course, is to make those financial barriers go away, but until the financial barriers are gone, the recognition that they are there allows me to deliver at least some beneficial care and hopefully not compromise the ideal too much. It is a stark reminder every day of the impact: the ludicrous realization that we spend tens of thousands of dollars on stents and bypass surgery and all this fancy stuff, and then we let them go, and for want of a few hundred bucks a year, all that work gets undone. It really defies any sense of logic.

JH: That is quite the story, and I am sure that has to be a tough conversation to have. For me, I never really knew my passion for medicine until I was already a medical student and I found this interest in upstream medicine through mentors, reading, community involvement, and classmates with similar interests. What drew you to medicine?

CS: I grew up in a really small rural town in New Brunswick. I guess what drew me to it was that it was intellectually challenging and it had a public-service appeal. It felt like a noble profession, and I found it exciting for all of those reasons. Just like nearly every medical student that gets into it, we go in with a fair bit of idealism, believing we are going to leave the world a better place than we found it. A lot of people talk about how that kind of idealism is beat out of students and residents. I have to confess it was probably beat out of me a bit in residency, but now it's back and better than ever before.

A lot of people say, "You are very Pollyanna-ish – everything is all roses and everything is positive," but if you do maintain that kind of idealism, it really can help you push through some of these tough issues. There is nothing wrong with having an aspirational goal, even if you recognize that we are never going to get there. The point is that we make progress toward that aspirational goal. That sort of positive view of the world is a very helpful way to approach a complex enterprise like medicine. It is something that I have tried to maintain, and I have found that it hasn't served me badly. When the social determinants came along, it just felt like the perfect fit. This is the thing that I was thinking about in more abstract terms as a medical student when I wanted to help people but didn't have a tangible sense of how. Then when I saw organized medicine and smart people actually developing tools to treat poverty and recognize the role of the doctor in doing things that can help health other than the delivery of healthcare and the practice of medicine, I found that so fascinating and so inspiring, it was just a natural fit.

▮▮ JH: I've heard you speak about how when you were in medical school you had a group of friends you used to get together with and talk about the future of medicine and how you were going to "leave the world a better place." Tell us a little bit about that.

▮▮ CS: It was a group of like-minded people who, early on in medical school, before really understanding the politics of medicine or the barriers in the profession, used to talk a lot about where we were going to be in twenty years, what we thought we were going to be doing. Then we would ask each other where we thought medicine was going to be and where public health was going to be – where is Canada going to rank internationally, and is medicare sustainable, all that kind of stuff. The tone was always very positive; nobody had a negative view of the future. Everybody said, "No, it's going to be better." There was this belief that everything was going to just continuously improve. Looking back twenty-five years, many things have improved, but there are a lot of things that haven't. Then there are some things that are exactly the same, the same old problems we are still talking about.

It is kind of interesting to reflect back on that and test our prognostic skills. Whether we have been successful or not in establishing change in our micro- or meso- or macro-environments is to me less important than the fact that we gave it our best effort. That is the role of the profession, to try to make our country and society a better place, and there are so many ways that you can do that. Some will succeed, some will succeed to a lesser degree, and some will fail and we will be wrong. The goals may be good, but the tactics we choose may be completely wrong. In those cases, we have to fail fast and try again. There is no role for the status quo for medicine and in health in Canada.

▮▮ Chapter 20 ▮▮

Expanding Perspective: A Geriatrician on Leadership, Time with Patients, and System Change

Samir Sinha (Advocate for Elder Care) – Marguerite Heyns

Dr Samir Sinha is a passionate and respected advocate for the needs of older adults. He currently works as director of geriatrics at Mount Sinai Hospital and the University Health Network Hospitals in Toronto. He is also assistant professor in the Departments of Medicine, Family and Community Medicine, and the Institute of Health Policy, Management and Evaluation at the University of Toronto, and assistant professor of medicine at the Johns Hopkins University School of Medicine. Prior to completing his residency in internal medicine, he won the Rhodes Scholarship, allowing him to complete a masters in medical history and a doctorate in sociology at Oxford. Dr Sinha's interdisciplinary background has allowed him to approach health policy and provision with a unique lens. During his tenure as the lead on Ontario's Seniors Strategy, he has significantly improved health outcomes for older adults in Ontario. More recently, he has been involved in the development of a National Seniors Strategy, making him one of the most compelling voices for the elderly in Canada.

When I met Dr Sinha for our interview, he was sitting halfway across the country in the community of Fort Albany in northern Ontario, part of a specialized care initiative focused on geriatric services for remote Indigenous communities. The program, North East Specialized Geriatric Services, provides upstream preventive care that addresses the root causes of poor health outcomes for the population it serves.

Naturally, his presence in Fort Albany flowed into our conversation and set the stage for the interview below.

■■ **Marguerite Heyns:** Medicine has been a part of my life plan since I was a kid. Like you, my father is also a physician, and he exposed me at a young age to the happiness and fulfillment his career afforded him. My dad has always deemed himself the luckiest man in the world because he has the privilege of helping people every day of his life for a living. He gets to impact people's lives, often when they are at their most vulnerable, for the better. The impact piece is really what stuck with me. This choice of profession is an opportunity for me to affect my community, society, and maybe even my country in a positive way. And that is why I'm here – it's what drives me to keep pushing through medical school, and it's also what helps me keep focused on what matters most: the patients. What was it that initially drew you to medicine?

■■ **Samir Sinha:** Children of healthcare professionals have had the privilege of being exposed. Growing up, both of my parents were physicians and many of our relatives were also physicians, and so we grew up in a medical household. You just knew that mom and dad would be home late because they were busy helping people. I think when my mom tried to explain to me what her job was as an obstetrician, she said, "I help the stork," and I thought that was pretty cool.

When I was a kid, every once in a while we would run into patients in the mall or out in the community and they would express their gratitude to my parents. Over time, medicine became very attractive to me. I grew up in a household that reminded me that with enormous privilege comes responsibility, and if you have the opportunity to help other people, medicine is a good way to do that. And from a very practical standpoint, medicine is also a very secure profession where you can also pursue a number of other interests, but people will always need healthcare providers.

MH: I know that you've done a masters and a PhD along with your MD. Where did those other degrees fall for you? Was medicine always the end goal?

SS: I did my graduate training after medical school. During my pre-med years, I had a real interest in having a very broad education, so I did English and geography and a bunch of other things that really expanded my thinking. It was in medical school that I got very interested in working with vulnerable populations in particular. My masters degree in history was actually a history of the care of the elderly in Britain from the founding of the National Health Service to present. And then my doctorate was an evaluation of the implementation of specific models of care of the elderly in England. The degrees are subtly misleading in thinking that they are complete departures. They were actually educational opportunities that allowed me to round out my knowledge and helped solidify my interest in working with the elderly. So I went from being interested in gastroenterology to being totally committed to a career in geriatrics.

MH: At the University of Calgary, where I study medicine, we have many mature students in our program, people that have had other careers or studied other disciplines, often in very diverse fields. And I think it's so exciting to think about what these people are going to do with medicine in the future.

SS: If you come in with a background, let's say English or sociology or international relations, you might bring a different perspective to medical school. But the challenge of medicine, especially in Canada, is

223

that once you come into medical school, you're not encouraged to do things beyond the usual program. You do your preclinical years, then you do your clinical years, then you go into residency, you get a job, and so on. In the US, medical schools are quite interesting because it's not uncommon for people to take a break between years two and three (between your preclinical and clinical part) and go off and do a masters and get extra training.

I found that medical school was really training you to be some kind of robot, a track that you get on and just do. Getting that opportunity to study in other fields after I'd gone through that whole machine, and then really learning about historical perspectives, policy, sociology, meant that when I came back into residency and thought about research and my career, I was much more determined and focused.

MH: I want to focus a bit on geriatrics and the specific population you work with. Almost serendipitously, we started our geriatrics unit in neurology this past week. It's something I have very much been looking forward to, because it's an area of health that poses some fairly big challenges for the future. In particular, I have been looking forward to learning about the innovations and strategies that will address the increased burden our ageing population threatens to impose on our healthcare system. What is the solution to the increasing costs we are already starting to face? Perhaps more importantly, how can we see this as an opportunity rather than a burden for our healthcare system?

SS: It's that classic story where older patients account for 15 per cent of our population, but account for 50 per cent of our healthcare cost. They are going to double over the next twenty years, and eighty-five-and-older people are going to quadruple, and that is where the bulk of healthcare spending is spent. So this population is going to bankrupt our country, and that's terrible. Our hospitals are full of frail elders. Their needs can't be adequately met, and our system is going to fail. So we keep hearing that as a huge challenge, and I certainly know all of the stats. I just reiterate them to make you scared about it, too. But I use that as an opportunity to get your attention and point out that this is a serious challenge. Then the question is, how do we actually create solutions?

There is a dearth of people who are doing work on geriatric models of care. Our current healthcare system was designed fifty years ago; the founding of medicare occurred when the average age of Canadians was twenty-seven. All of a sudden, we realize it made sense that our original system was about reimbursing physician services and hospital care. It had no concept of reimbursing long-term care, home care, in community care, or even medications. We didn't do any of those things because we didn't think those were essential elements.

We are now seeing that home community care costs $55 per day, long-term care costs $130 per day, but a day in hospital, where 7,500 older Canadians are living right now because they can't get any of those other services, costs $1,000 per day. Whether you are a staunch conservative or a left-leaning liberal, the point is there is an economic and humanistic justification to having a more elder-friendly approach to care. Care closer to home is not only cheaper, it's more in line with what people actually want.

The sad part is, we don't have enough people to do really pioneering work in this area given the support we currently have. The real focus should be on learning how to better care for older people or else they could bankrupt the system, while recognizing that the patients have changed and the system hasn't. I think with medical students, and with most professionals, the answers are there. They can come up with the answers, but we're not given the opportunity to recognize those problems and come up with solutions.

A lot of my work is around this. I like brainstorming with my colleagues to identify the problems, but more importantly to think of ways to make it better.

MH: What you're really talking about is a cultural shift in how we approach care of the elderly. Unfortunately that cultural shift hasn't occurred yet in the part of country where I'm learning how to practise medicine. So how can students like my colleagues and I be part of making that cultural shift happen?

SS: It's kind of like ostriches putting their heads in the sand. People are so overwhelmed, and they haven't been given the tools. Back to our medical education: we are widgets. Our training is also rooted in the way we created our healthcare system. It's all about curing, not about caring, and we're paid to act in that way as well. You're rewarded for seeing patients and doing tests, not for maintaining the sustainability of the healthcare system.

The challenges around geriatric care are that there are only 250 geriatricians in our county of 75,000 doctors. When you compare that to the care of children, there are over 1,500 pediatricians in the country, yet older people now outnumber younger people under fifteen. Students are not getting adequate exposure to the field. In neurology, for example, you will think of geriatrics from the dementia perspective, you will think about movement disorders, about Parkinson's, instead of thinking about broader concepts of frailty, or about functional and social issues.

MH: How does stigmatization affect the patients you work with?

SS: It's massive. People look at older patients and often they just see labels like dementia, and they think all of a sudden the patient is not even capable of making decisions. I always talk to my trainees about how labels kill. Be very careful which labels you ascribe to your patients because there is so much ageism, so much stigmatization of older patients that it could really end up impacting the care that they receive. One of my students was recently at another hospital in Toronto and asked his preceptor, "Do we have specific protocols around the care of elderly patients or patients with dementia?" and the guy said, "No, we don't bother doing that. We don't practise veterinary medicine." That's how he referred to patients with dementia, saying it's like dealing with animals, that you can't talk to them. My student was very upset and offended by that comment, because it just showed a complete disregard for the dignity and the need to actually be respectful and responsive to these patients' needs.

It's not uncommon to see ageism, which remains one of the last forms of accepted discrimination in our society. And that's not just discrimination against the old but also toward the youth. For some reason, ageism is permitted, while racism, sexism, whatever, are not. Somehow, making fun of older people, denying older people and younger people opportunities and supports is seen as okay. I think if we don't value growing old as a society, then we don't value the elderly; and if we don't value the elderly, why would we then value people who work with the elderly, or do care of the elderly? We don't prioritize geriatric training. For so long, geriatrics has remained this small, specialty group, largely because it was the lowest-paying medical specialty in the country. Who would want to do that? Who would want to take care of people that nobody cares about, and also take a pay cut?

We are actually not the lowest-paid specialty anymore, which is great, so that's no longer a barrier to people considering careers in geriatric medicine. We've really been focused on getting people to realize the value of geriatrics as well. The number one medical specialty in Britain is actually geriatric medicine. There are more geriatricians in Britain than cardiologists. In Canada, there are probably at least ten times as many cardiologists as there are geriatricians. It gives you a sense of how we value the elderly by how we as a country have chosen to prioritize our healthcare human resources.

MH: It sounds like things are changing, and that's maybe attracting more recent medical graduates to the specialty. And of course, you're doing lots of work on social media to bring public awareness to the profession. Are there any other ways you see this changing faster?

SS: I've been working on it with lots of colleagues behind the scenes. Our Canadian Medical Association represents 75,000 doctors, and what's the number one issue they are trying to focus on right now? A comprehensive seniors' strategy. When there are only 250 geriatricians, we can't be the only ones doing this.

Geriatrics is highly rewarding work, and you get to make huge impacts on the lives of older adults. Small things can actually make an enormous difference, and that's why geriatricians are the happiest physicians out there. Back to your father, who said, "I'm so privileged that I get to help people every day." When you see the level of help that you can bring to frail older patients when they have been so neglected by our healthcare system, how grateful they are, how rewarding it is to see how small things you can do can make an enormous difference, well, that's fantastic.

MH: I'm sure you have many patients that inspire you to continue the work that you do. Are there any particular stories that have stuck with you throughout your career?

SS: Geriatrics is a specialty that allows you to care for the entire patient. We can't get paid as geriatricians in Ontario unless we spend a minimum of ninety minutes with a patient. I do a lot of house calls, and you get to go meet people who've led the most incredible lives. I have patients who are former premiers of provinces and former captains of industry, people who've done the most interesting things. One of my patients built the Toronto subway system, and then he also built the Gardiner Expressway. It's cool when you have patients like these, and they come see you because they know how valuable you are at this point in their lives. They express that in many different ways in terms of how happy they are and how much they value coming to see you, which is a really lovely treat. We all like medicine because we all like to help people, but I think this is why geriatricians get to be some of the happiest people. We are doing work where not only do we know it's important, but these people know, too. After ninety years of living, they've never spent so much time with a doctor. We spend quite a bit of time listening to what's important, putting supports in place, and letting the person know you care.

MH: We have a lot of problems with access to care, especially for vulnerable and marginalized populations. Time is never something that comes up as a solution to reach more people and to really break down those barriers.

SS: People often think that something like spending time isn't really efficient, but when you take the time to untangle all of these complex problems, you get a huge payoff. I think people are starting to realize that the time and the comprehensive nature in which we do our care is actually a value-added investment. I think that's also why they've changed reimbursement for geriatricians, so it's not based on how many things you do but on the time that you spend with patients.

■■ MH: Canada is a country of migrants, many of them like me, immigrants or first-generation Canadians. Although that affords us an incredible amount of valuable diversity as a society, it also presents an increasingly common problem when we are considering care for our ageing population. Simply put, the traditional model of family support in old age just does not hold up in a modern Canada. To compound this issue further, our oldest folks are also living longer and often with more complex disabilities than ever before. How do you address the issue of under-supported patients, with families scattered across the country and around the world?

■■ SS: This is another common story. Compared to fifty years ago, we are less likely to be living in intergenerational households or communities. Traditional family networks are no longer the same either. When you look at the data, 28 per cent of Canadians report that they don't have a family member or friend close at hand who could help them with a basic task like getting a prescription filled. Older Canadians are leading more socially isolated lives than ever before, which actually impacts life expectancy, believe it or not. The question then is, how do you start changing things? With that in mind, a lot of the work that we are doing is looking at how we can ensure that we have adequate community care services. How can we make sure that we can help people rebuild their social networks, for example?

One thing we did in Ontario is look at the fact that one in three older adults suffers a fall on an annual basis. If an older person falls and fractures something, that costs the system a huge amount of dollars every year. In total, it costs Canada $2.2 billion annually to handle fractures in older adults. This means there's a huge interest in reducing falls, and there are things that we can do. In Ontario we funded $10 million in free exercise and falls-prevention classes for older adults. It's one of the things that I suggested to the government as part of the seniors' strategy. As a result, we also have people coming out to an activity where they can meet other older people and participate in a class. Maybe they make some friends and also start building a social network. Those 2,000 classes are offered only in publicly accessible locations throughout Ontario, and we had 170,000 older Ontarians participate in them last year. That's pretty cool, because while people may think of it as just being a health initiative to do exercise and falls-prevention classes, it's also a way to reduce social isolation.

MH: The last topic that I wanted to talk about is social determinants of health and how those affect the patients you are dealing with. How does your patients' access to things like income, food security, and housing impact your approach to medicine?

SS: The people geriatricians work with are often quite vulnerable and frail. What contributes to that? Well, if you're poor, you can't afford your medications; if you're poor, you can't afford transportation or food. These are the things that actually help maintain people's health and independence, especially at an older age. Talking about the complexity of these patients' care needs without addressing those social determinants of health – making sure people have adequate housing, transportation, basic income guarantees – is a major problem. One thing I always teach about in addition to the medical and functional issues is a third concept that I like to call social frailty. One of the big problems with social frailty is that when people don't have access to services or supports, it can really compromise their independence in the community. You can't do good geriatrics without assessing a patient's social situation and seeing whether they have risk factors that might limit them from leading healthy, independent lives.

■■ Chapter 21 ■■

Emergency Doctor by Choice, Defender of the Public Healthcare System by Necessity

Alain Vadeboncoeur (Médecins québecois pour le régime public) – Nina Nguyen

Long before my entry into medicine, Dr Vadeboncoeur was already established in Quebec media through TV, radio, and blogs. At sixteen, I was inspired by his sold-out play Sacré Coeur *("Sacred Heart") in Montreal in 2008. It was co-written with a playwright, and Dr Vadeboncoeur made sure the scenes, which mostly happened in an emergency room, were medically realistic. The result was a contemporary message that exposed the social role of the physician at the bedside of patients in distress that ended up at the ER as a last resort.*

It was by chance that I met Dr Vadeboncoeur through my involvement in medical student politics. Co-founder and past-president of Médecins québécois pour le régime public (MQRP), the Quebec equivalent of Canadian Doctors for Medicare, Dr Vadeboncoeur has always practised front-line medicine. He believes that access to care is one of the social determinants of health over which physicians have the most control.

Bringing together around five hundred members from all levels of medical practice, including medical students, MQRP sets itself apart as the medical professional voice that defends the public healthcare system.

Dr Vadeboncoeur has been based at the Montreal Heart Institute (Institut de cardiologie de Montréal) since 1999, where he is currently the head of the Emergency Medicine Department. I met

with Dr Vadeboncoeur there to discuss the civic engagement that frames his medical practice, mixing emergency medicine, teaching, research, and health communication.

■■ **Nina Nguyen:** Tackling the social determinants of health in medicine seems to be a recent line of thought, and it is usually family doctors who are involved. As an emergency doctor, how do you see the consequences of the social determinants of health in your patients?

■■ **Alain Vadeboncoeur:** The emergency ward is a universal greeting room for human distress. Social crises, which often have psychological and physical components, often end up at the emergency room, where patients in distress end up because they have nowhere else to turn. The "frequent flyers" of the emergency room are often people who have fewer resources and unresolved social issues, and do not have the ability to navigate the healthcare system. The emergency room becomes a kind of magnet toward which patients are attracted – at least, we hope – so that we can help them even though it might not be the most appropriate setting. So the emergency room is somewhat of a concentrated version of society.

At Pierre-Boucher Hospital, there were "frequent flyers" who lived in a nearby rooming house for people with difficulties. These people were suffering from extreme poverty, had no job, and often had no resources and no social networks. Sometimes, we are their social networks, because they would have been lonely otherwise. For me, the emergency room is really a mirror, a reflection of the society in general, including its difficulties, and every crisis goes through it. It is one of the best places to examine what is going well or not in our society.

■■ **NN:** As an emergency doctor, have you had occasion to address these determinants of health in your practice?

AV: From the point of view of the emergency room, it is obvious that continuity of care is lacking. We have one-time meetings with people, sometimes in distress, who will be admitted or leave. It is relatively easy to identify social determinants, and I would even say it is a context where we can influence these determinants.

Once we have identified an issue, it is at that moment that teams and links with external resources will help us. For example, if I have an elderly patient who is visibly in distress because it is not working well at home anymore, hopefully there are other professionals who will step in. The network nurse, the social workers, they are now working in all emergency departments. It is through these teams that we are able to manage a social risk that will influence the health of the patient.

Of course, the emergency room is much more of a diagnostic setting, and I don't have much expertise in managing these complex issues, but I am at least able to direct them to professionals who are more qualified than I. That's an important part of my job.

NN: I find it interesting that you say you are not that much involved in case management when meeting the media or when taking care of patients, but for you, it is really that involvement outside of work that helps you "catch up" on that side of medicine.

AV: Are you saying I should feel guilty? [Laughs.] No, but at the same time, it probably stems from my experience in the emergency room.

In the emergency room, there is one criterion: if you are dying, you will be seen before the other patients, and nothing else matters. In hospitals, there are very wealthy people who come to the emergency room, for example the hospital's great donors. It is still obvious that the clinical condition should come first, and it's even truer in the emergency room than anywhere else. My practice already leads me to identify the most urgent needs and to take care of them. It is as simple as that; once the patients are in hospital gowns, they are not that different from one another. That's why MQRP's logo is a hospital gown. It's a symbol that the health system should be egalitarian.

So I treat people 100 per cent accordingly to their needs, and in a context that they all have access to care, without question. Even patients without a health card, here we don't care about it, and that's true for anywhere. It's not because we are particularly virtuous, we just won't discriminate against a patient with a heart infarction; you can't do that!

Maybe that is what has influenced me to a certain extent, and gives me this vision, shared by a lot of people, of a healthcare system for all.

■■ **NN:** What prompted you to start MQRP?

■■ **AV:** It's important to know that MQRP was started in 2008, but it already existed previously under another name, Doctors for Access. That started in 2005 and had the mission to respond to the Chaoulli ruling of the Quebec Supreme Court that removed the ban on private health insurance for care and services offered by medicare. I was really interested in healthcare from the emergency perspective. I also saw that the important questions weren't always being asked as they should. Attending a Doctors for Access meeting further sparked my interest in the topic, and I set out to learn more.

Doctors for Access was working well as an organization, but it wasn't consistent or well structured. A group of us decided to reorganize it. At the beginning, the idea was access, with no prejudice against the private or the public healthcare system per se. It was more like a scientific analysis of reality, and if we saw that the private sector would be more successful, why not? One of the first discussions was what to call ourselves; we needed a good name. Were we going to side with the public system? In the end, the private sector grows by itself, it is the public sector that is threatened, and it is the public sector that is the main determining factor for access. So we agreed to add it to our name, so we could make the identity of the organization stronger.

It is not enough that we were stressing better access; we also wanted to defend the public system, which is the main determining factor of access in the end. There were no doctors who were speaking up, and there was no organization in Quebec that was doing so. We wanted to build a real organization with a general assembly and a real democratic process, with an executive board, and this is what happened.

MQRP has brought up many issues that were not often discussed before. Now there is a medical voice. What I find most fascinating is the resonance within students, young doctors, and medical residents alike. Yes, it might fit with the values of these groups much more than those of the doctors over sixty years old who have been practising for a while. I find students more sensitive to these issues than doctors of my own generation. That being said, back in my time, there were also people who were aware. It is almost like doctors distance themselves from these issues over time, because most of the doctors are usually aware in a general sense. I'm not sure exactly what phenomenon causes them to lose sight of this.

French version available at - http://hdl.handle.net/2429/60457

▪▪ Afterword ▪▪

Dr Jeff Turnbull

Equity is an essential principle of social justice and something that is often referred to as part of the Canadian identity. As a goal, health equity requires that all within Canada have the opportunity to achieve their full health potential regardless of who they are, where they live, or what they have.

Invariably, this draws us into a consideration of the broader societal factors that influence our health beyond that of the healthcare system, such as ethnicity, gender and sexual orientation, poverty, language, education, housing, and location, to name a few. Equity within the healthcare system, whether it relates to access, experience, or outcomes, has the opportunity to mitigate many of these social variables in a fair and just society.

As a wealthy and technologically advanced country, we have become obsessed with the allure of robotics, proteomics, and genomics, while remaining blind to disadvantaged communities throughout Canada that experience health outcomes comparable to those of the poorest countries in the developing world. In my practice with Ottawa's homeless, I see the prevalence and severity of illness as bad as or worse than any place I have been in Africa or Southeast Asia. I see daily the consequences of poverty, marginalization, inadequate early childhood development, lack of education, and unemployment, all compounded by mental illness and addictions. This is a heavy price for individuals to pay for their misfortune, but also for us as a society. To fail to advocate against this social inequity and its causes is a failure of our profession.

Who better then to bring us back to the roots of our profession than our future doctors? The remarkable medical students and residents who conducted the interviews in this collection relate their struggles in keeping up with the advances of modern medicine while refocusing their attention on the social determinants of health, which in the end are more powerful in influencing health outcomes. Through their narratives, key medical leaders and social justice advocates describe their perception of health and healthcare within Canada, the challenges in moving us forward, and what brought them to address the social determinants of health through upstream strategies. Within each story of individual insight and dedication is a rich dialogue highlighting the importance of revisiting the fundamental values of medicine, such as advocacy, service, compassion, professionalism, and caring.

In reading this collection of interviews, one cannot help but think that modern medicine has lost its way and that we are now being shown a new path by those who follow. If the future of medicine is in the hands of these distinguished physicians and the remarkable medical students interviewing them, then we have every reason for optimism.

■■ Editors' Biographies ■■

■■ **Andrew Bresnahan** is an anthropologist and resident physician in the Northern Family Medicine Program based in Labrador, Canada, and past vice-president, Global Health of the Canadian Federation of Medical Students.

■■ **Mahli Brindamour** is a general pediatrician working in Saskatoon with a special interest in refugee health and Northern health.

■■ **Christopher Charles** is a resident physician in anesthesiologyin Toronto, inventor and founder of the *Lucky Iron Fish Project*, and past vice-president, Global Health of the Canadian Federation of Medical Students.

■■ **Ryan Meili** is a family physician in inner-city Saskatoon, founder of Upstream, and author of *A Healthy Society: How a Focus on Health can Revive Canadian Democracy.*